“I’ve Tried It All! Now What?!”

The New Rules for Diet Dropouts

Susanna H. Wermuth

"I've Tried It All! Now What?!"

Susanna H. Wermuth

Published by:
Top Shelf Books
a division of Jawbone Publishing Corp.
2907 Paddington Way
Kissimmee, FL 34747
marketing@jawbonepublishing.com
http://www.jawbonepublishing.com

Author Contact Information:
Susanna H. Wermuth
P.O. Box 752
Gotha, FL 34734
sw@dietdropouts.com
http://www.dietdropouts.com

Printed in the United States of America.

This one's for me

Table of Contents

PART I

"I've Tried It All! Now What?!"

Real People are Diet Dropouts

When is somebody going to stand up and scream, "NONE OF THIS WORKS!!!!"? Who is going to indignantly proclaim, "YOU'VE GOT TO BE KIDDING!!!!!"? When is someone going to just slap the Versace suit off of that "expert" giving us weight loss advice on *The View*? And who is going to have the guts to tell Dr. Phil he doesn't have the ultimate weight loss solution?!

All of us, including Dr. Phil, need to get real! Let's face it, real people (*aka: the majority of the population*) don't make "healthy lifestyle changes". Real people don't want to give up their bacon cheeseburgers. Real people aren't going to head for the gym after they've been told the accounting firm taking care of their business is facing fraud charges. Real people don't grab a rice cake when they've found out what their 16-year-old daughter was really doing at her friend's house last night. Real people don't want to eat 3 cantaloupes and 11 stalks of celery instead of a piece of white-chocolate-raspberry cheesecake.

Real people ***do*** want to grab a piece of pizza and a soda for lunch. Real people want to go out and enjoy a meal with good friends and good wine, instead of counting the calories, carbohydrates, fat grams, percentages, and/or points they have left to eat in a day. Real people often "drive through" to get dinner rather than facing the prospect of actually *making* dinner and cleaning dishes *in addition to* doing laundry, bathing the kids, making sure homework is done, returning phone calls, etc. etc..

When real people do try to commit to a diet and/or exercise program, their resolve is short-lived. On those rare occasions when real people do muster up every ounce of their willpower and lose weight, they regain it quickly along with a few extra pounds for bad measure. In short, real people are diet drop-outs.

The statistics regarding real people and weight loss prove the diet and exercise industry has failed and continues to fail us miserably. But here's the good news: We can and must look elsewhere for the answers. That brings us to this book. So go grab a highlighter pen and get ready to mark up theses pages! You are required to review and re-review those highlighted areas which make so much more common sense than anything you have read before about weight loss.

Okay, that said, this book is a sitting duck, no doubt about it. At this very moment, there are advocates and professionals in the diet, exercise, and medical industries who are taking shots at what I have written here with their volumes of data on the benefits of diet and exercise. You may even encounter some reservations of your own. However, this book does not, at any point, try to disclaim those benefits.

For the most part, there is no arguing the scientific findings which overflow in the myriad of diet and exercise books that sit right next to this one on the shelf of your local bookstore. And let us not forget the almost daily barrage of information we can find on the newsstand, television, and internet.

There is no debating that exercise builds muscle and muscle burns fat. There is no debating that there are 0 fat grams in lettuce and plenty of fat grams in a cheeseburger. Everyone knows exercise burns calories and there are more calories in a brownie than there is in a carrot. And there are very few people who haven't heard exercise increases your metabolism and a faster metabolism burns more calories, etc. etc..

I think it's safe to assume most people know at least the basic workings and benefits of eating healthy foods and exercising – how could they not? The question this book addresses is why can't the majority of those same people lose weight and keep it off?

The answer is very simple but will go against every grain of information we have allowed the diet and exercise industry to instill in our psyches. Aside from the individual who has a legitimate health problem, ***a person does not have to exercise, diet, take drugs, or make a lifetime commitment to a healthy lifestyle to lose weight.***

Not that exercising isn't healthy for you, or that eating low fat foods won't lower your cholesterol levels - no one is debating that. But you do not *have to* do either to lose weight and stay thin. In fact - *now hold on to your seatbelts* - there are many cases, like mine, where diet and exercise are primarily responsible for the weight gain in the first place. But more about that later.

This would be a good time to remind anyone who does want to lose weight to consult with their physician before embarking on any weight loss program. I am not a physician, but I'll be honest, nothing my physician had to say helped me lose the 65 pounds I needed to lose. "Cut your calories and exercise," I remember him saying. My unspoken reply was, 'Tell me something I don't know!'

But what I also know now is I went from a size 18 to a size 4, eating anything, any time, and without a lick of exercise. More importantly, I have been a size 4 for over 15 years even though I have had plenty of reasons to have regained the weight. I became a mother, went through a messy divorce and custody battle, and I turned the two ages that are most credited for the middle-age spread.

During those same 15 years, I have watched the majority of the population embrace diet book after diet book, exercise machine after exercise machine, magic pill after magic pill, only to become fatter and fatter. Before that time, I had never imagined getting close to a size 4 especially since I am over 5'7" tall. My goal was to fit back into my size 9 jeans (*a pretty ambitious goal to begin with*), but I wound up at a model's weight. And may I say again, I have been a size 4 for over 15 years. Fortunately, that's the one thing my critics can't argue with - undeniable success.

Ironically, my struggle with weight loss began when I was looking to lose a mere 3 pounds. I was 17 years old and a senior in high school. From the time I was six, I was involved in the competitive world of ice skating, but by my senior year, my ice skating career was winding down. I was gaining more interest in school and its extra-curricular activities, not the least of which was returning the flirtation of high school boys.

Throughout the time I spent ice skating, I had observed many of my competitors obsessing about their weight. They would try just about anything to lose the 2 or 3 or 15 pounds their coaches insisted they lose. There was always some skater in our group who was on the newest fad diet.

I'll never forget a particular incident I witnessed at a party that my skating coach was hosting at her beach house. While most of the partygoers were on the beach, one of my coach's other skaters and I went back to the beach house to go to the bathroom. When I was finished with my turn in the powder room, I walked out and I found the other girl in the kitchen, spooning heaps of peanut butter on lettuce and ravenously gobbling it down.

I didn't say anything because I was a little taken aback by her odd behavior. I knew she was desperately trying to lose weight and I was fairly sure a half jar of peanut butter was not on the diet. At the time, I had never really thought much about dieting myself, or food at all for that matter, so it was easy for me to be slightly judgmental about the situation. Little did I know, a year or two later I would be caught up in my own diet hell and exhibiting the same odd behavior.

By the fall of my senior year, I was only skating occasionally. *(Please resist the temptation of thinking what you have been programmed to think – that I started gaining weight because I was less active - you would be wrong.)* But for the first time, I was attracting the attention of the young men in my class. Even though it was thrilling, it was a little confusing because I had never ever attracted this much attention ever! All I knew is I loved it, and I wanted to hang on to it!

So when I looked in the mirror one day and noticed that my jeans had become a little tight, I panicked. It could have very well been that certain time of the month when every woman retains a little water, but that's not what I was thinking. What I was thinking is that certainly one of the reasons I was attracting the boys was because I was thin.

I needed to make sure I stayed thin, so logically I decided to go on a diet to lose 3 pounds. *Easy.* I grabbed a magazine off the newsstand that promised, "Lose 5 Pounds in 3 Days!" I looked at the diet plan. It not only spelled out exactly what to eat and drink and at what time, but it measured out everything for you! It couldn't get any easier! I naively resolved to myself, *"I'll start tomorrow."*

".....I'll start tomorrow." - The powerfully negative implications that lurked behind those 3 simple words wouldn't become apparent to me until many years later. But, with those words in mind and on the eve of my first diet, I indulged myself with an extra large piece of cake for dessert. 'After all,' I thought, 'I won't be able to have cake for the next 3 days.' I went to bed with a bit of a stomach ache, but was much comforted by the thought that I would be 5 pounds thinner in just 3 days!

Do I even have to tell you how this story ends? Probably not, because chances are this is your story too. The details may be different, but the story is the same. Whether it was 3 pounds or 300 pounds, whether it was "5 Pounds in 3 Days" or a seemingly healthier plan like "Weight Watchers", and whether it was an extra large piece of cake or a whole month or year of overeating before the onset of the next diet and exercise regimen, the dynamics are the same.

I know because I replayed this story over and over and over, always with more weight to lose and a different program that I would "start tomorrow". But no matter the circumstances, the story always wound up the same - I would fall off the program and quickly gain back all the lost weight and more.

A few years later, I was 65 pounds heavier, and absolutely miserable. Not only did my body feel heavy, my mind and spirit were suffocating from the weight. I thought about food constantly - what I should eat, what I shouldn't eat, when I should eat, when I shouldn't eat, how much I should eat, how I ate too much, how I have to stop eating, what food I couldn't resist and how weak I was for not being able to resist it.

I would spend hours exercising - at one point running 4 miles a day - only to see the weight creep back on to my body with a vengeance. Many an evening, I would lay in my bed, with silent tears streaming down my face and calling out to God for help, but my agonizing plight continued.

During that time, I avoided cameras like the plague. Out of the few pictures that were taken, I only saved one and that is the one you see here on the back cover of this book. Looking at that picture now, I'd like to say I was fat because I was a young woman dealing with self-esteem issues because of her somewhat dysfunctional childhood. Although the latter would be true, unlike the popular psychology doled out today by people like Dr. Phil, the realization of my emotional dysfunction and working on my "issues" did not lead to my ultimate weight loss.

In fact, it wasn't until 10 years later after I had lost all my weight I started working on those issues. And I have to admit I'm still working on them, but that's another book. What's interesting is that if Dr. Phil sat me down at that particular point in my life, he could have easily convinced me my father's absence, my mother's behavior, or my grandmother's death was the cause for my overeating.

The wonderful thing about my weight loss story and the basis of my weight loss consulting business is you will find no mention of psychotherapy. Nor will you find mention of willpower or making commitments to drugs, diet, exercise, or healthy lifestyles.

Instead, the most enormous obstacle any of my clients have had to overcome is how very, very, very, simple losing weight can be with the New Rules. So simple, I can tell in my first consultation with a client if they are still not ready for how simple it is.

Some clients are still convinced there is a "diet" or some other form of laborious program that is the key to their weight loss. Some are actually frightened at the thought of not relying on a program. I tell them to come back to me after they've tried a few more diets and a few more unused memberships at the gym.

And if you read this book and you too decide it can't be this simple or you too are frightened at the thought of being regimen-free, keep this book on a shelf somewhere close. After a few years and a few more programs and no doubt, a whole lot more money spent and weight regained, blow the dust off its pages, and reread it.

In our present and future world of unprecedented knowledge and technology, the simplest things will continue to become the hardest to realize. My hope is that you are ready to relax, absorb, and then implement this very simple concept with the help of these very simple rules.

Knowing More, Spending More, But Weighing More

I went to an internet bookstore today and typed in the words "diet and fitness" in the search box. *Guess how many books they were offering in this category? .... No go ahead and take a wild guess......... 100? 200? 500?* Nope. My search came up with 30,111 results – **30,111** books on diet and fitness!

Go browsing on the rest of the World Wide Web and your searches will come up with additional tens and hundreds of thousands of results when you inquire about diet, fitness, and weight loss. And almost daily there are new facts and figures to be added to the subject.

Clearly, there has never been a time in history that we've known more information about how a fat, calorie, sugar, fiber, or carbohydrate is processed in our bodies. Never before in history have we been so inundated with knowledge about the different muscles, bones, and organs in our bodies - what they do, how they do it, how to build them, and what to feed them.

Never has there been a time when more money has been spent in researching, developing, and producing drugs to aid us in losing weight, or a time we have spent more money on diet and fitness products. ***And there has never been a time in history we have been fatter!*** It doesn't take an art aficionado to figure out there is something desperately wrong with this picture.

America's waistline isn't the only thing that is expanding – almost in direct correlation is the expanding wallet of the weight loss industry. As of this printing it is estimated that Americans currently spend $40 - $50 billion a year on the battle of the bulge. Corporate America circles the science of weight loss like vultures. They can hardly wait for the next tidbit of research that will produce a new drug, product, or program upon which to capitalize.

In the mid-1990's, a very powerful and popular American company which specializes in cookies and snacks made a fortune on the low-fat trend. The newest science of the time was touting the theory of losing fat by not ingesting fat. Books upon books were being written about the latest findings about how a fat calorie is processed differently than a carbohydrate or protein calorie. Promises of extraordinary weight loss were being made to those who would start counting fat grams and keep them to a minimum.

This company quickly jumped on the capitalistic bandwagon by producing a line of low-fat and non-fat cookies. They hit the mother load. The demand for a particular non-fat cookie reached such a fevered pitch the product had to be rationed to grocery stores! There was an almost surreal public response - fighting in the grocery aisles, groups formed to anticipate delivery of the cookies, and cookies being put under lock and key.

Regardless, the craze passed just as the many crazes that preceded it and for the same reason - after a few years of eating the cookies, consumers weighed more, not less. Why? Because all the company did was replace fat calories with sugar calories, barely changing the caloric intake.

However, Americans weren't the only ones

"pigging out". The company was feeding on the public's new belief that since they were consuming no fat grams, they could eat as many cookies as they wanted without suffering any consequences. Millions of cookies were sold.

Make no mistake though, even though results clearly suggest otherwise, the messages linking low-fat and non-fat products to weight loss have been branded into the American psyche as if it were unquestionable scientific fact. LOW FAT, NON FAT, and REDUCED FAT are still words the food industry continues to cash in on. Just stroll down the aisles of your local grocery store and you will be hard pressed to find an item which doesn't have a lower fat version placed next to it.

So what's wrong with ingesting less fat? *Absolutely nothing. If you are trying to lower your cholesterol and make healthier choices – great.* But that's not what the industry is banking on. The industry is banking on what the majority of overweight consumers tend to think, whether consciously or more often unconsciously. 'Well, there's less fat in this so I can eat more of it.' The more you eat, the more they sell. The more you eat, the more you weigh. The more you weigh, the more you will be looking for more low-fat products.

Additionally, consumers forget fat is one of the key components which satisfies our physical hunger. Less fat means it will take more of a certain product to reach a person's satiety level, the point where an individual feels satisfied. Again, this means more low-fat food sold, more low-fat food eaten, and more pounds gained. Admittedly, it's a sound business plan – one that perpetuates demand. But this Catch-22 is solely at your expense – financially, mentally, and physically.

Then there are the weight loss programs. Some are now virtually extinct such as Nutri-System, but there are others like Weight Watchers and Jenny Craig who have and continue to enjoy a very long and successful run in the industry. But when I refer to successful I'm referring to the company's financial success, not their clients' weight loss successes.

In fact, no weight loss company has been really forthcoming with their clients' long term success rates. Why? Some companies claim it is too costly to track their clients. *(Funny, you would think that high success rates would be worth their weight in gold in promoting their program.)* Others will say that up to 95% of their clients lose weight on their program, but dodge the questions of how much weight and how long they keep it off. The truth is companies guard this information as if it was a matter of national security because if their clients really knew the facts, they would be out of business.

What are the facts? Well, diets do work. Any weight loss diet that you follow to the letter will result in lost weight. I could make one up right here, right now, and if you ate only what I told you to eat you would lose weight, but that's not the problem. The problem is what happens after the diet. Studies vary, but it's estimated that as few as 4 out of every 1000 dieters maintain their weight loss for any significant period of time. The other 946 gain all their weight back and often times more. That is a success rate of 0.4%! Can you imagine any other business that would be able to stay in business with a success rate of less than 1%?

The more financially successful programs, however, have made good use of the psychology of dieting to create a dependency on their services. When you follow their program, you indeed lose weight. When you fall off their program, you gain weight. You go back to their program, and lose weight again. You go off their program and gain the weight back again.

Conclusion: They are responsible for getting you thin and you are responsible for getting fat. That means you cannot do it without them. You must surrender your power (and money) to them to stay thin. They, of course, know the statistics. They know you will fall off the program, regain the weight, and need them again. It's another one of those Catch-22s - sound business, but at your expense.

Government agencies are finally, however slowly, starting to crack down on the diet industry. They have not been able to get the industry to produce legitimate success rates because apparently the definition of "success" is highly debatable. But they have managed to get companies to publish disclaimers in their advertising. You know, those teeny tiny words that flash across the screen of a commercial that you need a magnifying glass to read: *Results not typical.* I had to laugh the first time I saw, *Results atypical,* clearly intended for those with good eyesight but not necessarily avid readers of Webster's Collegiate Dictionary.

The bottom line is that all these members of the weight loss industry are taking your money, leaving disastrous results in their wake. The most recent figures from the National Center for Chronic Disease Prevention and Health Promotion show that from 1991 – 2000, the number of overweight adult Americans has increased by a whopping 61% with no downward trend in sight.

Statistics also show that 64.5% of Americans

are now overweight and approximately 25% of adults are so overweight they can be described as "obese". Weight trends for our children are just as disturbing with obesity rates doubling in children and tripling in adolescents since 1980. The CDC has gone as far as declaring obesity an "epidemic" in our country directly resulting in the increase of obesity-related diseases such heart disease and diabetes.

The far reaching effects of obesity to our nation's healthcare system have the Senate Committee on Health, Education, Labor and Pensions desperately looking for solutions to the problem. Experts testifying before the Committee are placing blame on the decrease of activity and the increase of fast food consumption in our society. They are also asking for government involvement to get Americans moving more and eating healthier.

All I have to say is *good luck*. Americans have been incessantly told over the last few decades that they should be exercising more and eating vegetables instead of Big Macs. Nine out of every ten magazines we see on the newsstands have at least one article discussing what we should be doing to lose weight.

Every news show on television has spent their share of time devoted to nutrition, weight loss, and exercise tips. Rarely does a half an hour go by, without a commercial touting a low-fat or diet product. We can't get in our car and turn on the radio without hearing why we should join Bally's or Gold's Gym. When we do turn off the radio, there's always a billboard to drive by showing a before and after picture of some person who has eaten low-fat sub sandwiches to lose their weight.

Oh, there's no doubt that Americans know what

they supposedly "should" be doing. The mystery is why isn't it working?

Oprah: Don't Make the Connection
Break the Connection

Who hasn't watched the very public weight loss roller coaster Oprah has been on for the last 16 years? As most overweight people know, it is hard enough to deal with the problem of weight loss and regain on a personal level, but to see it chronicled almost daily on national television takes a very strong individual.

I suppose that same strength is what allowed Oprah to go on a diet called OptiFast in July of 1988 – a 4-month liquid regimen which could be considered almost inhumane. In November of 1988, Oprah dedicated one of her shows to discussing her dramatic weight loss experienced through OptiFast. Immediately after the telecast, sales for the company soared …. unfortunately so did Oprah's weight.

In the book, *Make the Connection*, Oprah described the horror as her weight almost instantaneously began to climb back up after the liquid fast. Entries in her journal written just 2 weeks after she declared her success to the world show an intimate look into a dieter's hell; bingeing, panic, guilt, self-loathing, and an unnatural obsession with her scale.

Ironically, just 5 months before Oprah's fast, I had written her a letter about this new discovery of mine which still did not have a name. The many times when she had talked about food and dieting on her show sounded so much like my experience I thought the New Rules could truly help her as they had helped me.

Less than 8 weeks later Oprah personally wrote me back. A copy of the actual letter is the one you see below – obviously written at a time when her celebrity was not so enormous she could not personally answer my letter. But it was also written when she was still looking for yet another diet which would work for her.

Unfortunately, Oprah did not contact me after the failure of the "plan of [her] own". Less than 4 years and some other unsuccessful diets later, Oprah was at her highest weight ever. About that time she met a personal trainer with whom she is still presently associated, Bob Greene.

The Oprah Winfrey Show

P.O. BOX 909715, CHICAGO, ILLINOIS 60690

Apr 28, 1988

Dear Susanna,

Thanks so much for your offer to help me with my diet. I'm currently trying a plan of my own though. But--if it doesn't work out, I'll have your letter on file.

Best wishes,

Oprah Winfrey

In March 1993, Greene started Oprah on a vigorous exercise program and a healthy eating plan. Oprah had to give up most of her favorite foods and worked up to running 8 miles a day, admittedly hating most every minute of it. Eight months later, she had lost 72 pounds and was ready to run in her first marathon.

Shortly after the marathon, Oprah again dedicated one of her shows to her newly found weight loss, explaining that she had finally "made the connection". She explained it wasn't about losing weight and dieting but just consciously choosing to do what's best for yourself and your body each day. Oprah so much as said this "connection" was the end of her issues with weight.

Fittingly enough, Bob Greene sat next to her that day touting his new book called *Make the Connection.* And just as Oprah had done with her low-fat chef, Rosie, years before, she made Greene a best-selling author overnight. Greene's program, however, did not end Oprah's issues with weight because it was still basically a diet and exercise regimen.

For the next ten years, Oprah's weight continued to fluctuate despite the many other diet and fitness authors she spotlighted on her show. She also had many psychologists join her on the show to help her work through her "issues" regarding her weight, but again nothing took her off the weight loss roller coaster.

More recently Oprah announced again on a show dedicated to weight loss that she has finally 'got it'. With Bob Greene still by her side with yet another new book, Oprah excitedly pronounced, "Diets don't work!" She and Greene continued with that theme pointing out, quite correctly, diets only set you up for failure.

I thought to myself, 'Could this be it? Did she finally figure out what I had over 15 years ago?' But it didn't take long to see the whole show just put a different spin on what is still essentially a diet and exercise program which Oprah has implemented in her life. True, it was a little less stringent, but still highly unrealistic for a real person to incorporate.

My mouth fell wide open when Oprah read the contract which Greene had her sign 6 weeks before the Emmys. The agreement was obviously designed to get her in shape in time for the event. The contract included things like committing to an hour of intense exercise 6 days a week and choosing foods for nutritional rather than emotional reasons. It also restricted alcohol of any kind for 6 weeks and had an agreement to not eat anything 2 hours prior to bedtime.

If that wasn't bad enough, there was a clause in the contract where Oprah had to acknowledge her failure in the past to committing to any similar programs. Then she also had to acknowledge the contract was only with herself and carried no rewards or punishments EXCEPT any that might be associated with the reflection of the strength of her character!

......NO REWARDS OR PENALTIES EXCEPT FOR ANY THAT MIGHT BE ASSOCIATED WITH THE REFLECTION OF THE STRENGTH OF HER CHARACTER?????? OH....MY....GOD!!!! *And that couldn't possibly be setting her up for failure like an ordinary diet????* I was AGHAST!!!!

Then Oprah went on to say how she called Greene up during that period of time and literally begged him to allow her a single glass of champagne at a party held in her honor. He verbally threw the contract back in her face and she did not have the champagne. I COULD NOT BELIEVE MY EARS!!! It was enough to make me run to the kitchen and grab a glass of wine and a handful of potato chips!!!

Of course Oprah looked great at the Emmys, but at what cost? Once you understand the New Rules, you will understand the very damaging and long term effects that contract will wield in Oprah's life - not to mention in the lives of the millions of viewers who watch Oprah's show.

And I will lay good money on the fact that Oprah's weight will continue to yo-yo in the years to come. How do I know? Let me answer that: ***Because Oprah is a real person who loves macaroni and cheese and hates to exercise!!!!!*** This is not rocket science!

So you might be thinking about now, if Oprah, with all her money, personal trainers, personal chefs, therapists, and all her other resources, can't achieve permanent weight loss, how am I? Let me answer that too - real people like you and Oprah will achieve permanent weight loss by breaking, *not making*, the connection of exercise and healthy eating to weight loss.

As I have said before, there is no debating the health benefits of exercise and eating healthy foods, but you do not have to do either to lose weight permanently. *Pretty scandalous statement, isn't it?* But it's true.

Emancipating the Diet Slaves

There is no doubt you can lose weight as Oprah did, by exercising and eating healthily, but rarely is it permanent for the same reasons other less healthier weight loss programs don't work long term. ***Weight loss programs take away your personal choices***.

It's a lot easier to see how this is true with an extreme program like OptiFast, where you only drink vitamin shakes all day, every day for weeks or months at a time. Obviously, your choices have been taken away - what you will eat, when you will eat, and how much you will eat.

But the fact is *any* weight loss program, including the seemingly sane one which Bob Greene implemented for Oprah, essentially takes away some or all of your personal choices. You give up at least one of the following: what to eat, when to eat it, and how much to eat in order to lose weight.

The same goes for exercise - how to exercise, when to exercise, and how much to exercise in order to shed those pounds. If you are a real person, even the more general version of "exercise and eat healthy foods" strongly implies the only way you're going to lose the weight is if you're willing to give up your lifestyle choices and the foods you love.

What essentially are we when we've given up our personal choices? We are slaves. We have traded our most basic human rights of eating and moving for a 0.4% chance of permanent weight loss.

And what happens when you enslave someone? It stirs up resentment and anger within them.

They eventually rebel because the necessity for freedom is part of the human psyche. When you challenge part of the human psyche, you are dealing with something very powerful and you will get a powerful response. It is what has fueled human and civil rights movements and even started wars throughout history. This is why dieters, shortly after beginning a new program, start feeling resentful and angry. It's a basic human response when our freedoms are infringed upon.

When resentment and anger turns to rebellion, history also shows us it can be violent. The Berlin Wall was taken down easily by human hands! Dieters are no different. When dieters take their freedom back, they go on a rampage, eating everything they weren't allowed to eat and as much as they want to eat! They stop running those 5 miles a day and sit on the couch watching TV instead.

Another powerful force dieters have working against them is what humans share with every living thing - survival. ***Our bodies are built to avoid deprivation and pain.***

Dieting of any kind is deprivation. This is more obvious when we are speaking simply in terms of shortage or lack of food. It is less obvious when we see commercially successful diets address the issue of deprivation by claiming you can eat a "limitless" or an "enormous" amount of a particular food so you will never feel hungry. But the feeling of fullness is only one small factor of the satiety equation.

Let's say you are really craving macaroni and cheese, but you are not allowed to have it on your new weight loss plan. Instead you eat something "legal" or "free" like a huge bowl of steamed green beans,

4 slices of cantaloupe, and a grilled piece of fish. You can still feel a profound sense of deprivation and even hunger although your stomach is physically stuffed because you did not satisfy the initial craving. Either way, we are deprived. ***Dieting equals deprivation.***

Exercise, respectively, is a form of pain and exertion. How many times have you heard the expression, "No pain, no gain," in relationship to an exercise program? Unfortunately, humans were built to avoid pain, not to inflict it upon themselves. From the time the wheel was invented to the more recent innovations of computer technology, mankind has looked for ways to make life and work less painful, not more painful. ***Exercise essentially equals pain.***

So here we have a multi-billion dollar industry sending us constant messages that the only way to lose weight is through slavery, deprivation, and pain – going against our most innate human mechanisms. Worse yet, we are faced with a lifetime of slavery, deprivation, and pain – oftentimes masked under the euphemistic phrase "making a healthy lifestyle change" - to maintain the weight loss! Is it any wonder the weight loss industry has failed us miserably and has even contributed to the problem?

The solution lies in emancipating the diet slaves - but wisely and gently. When President Lincoln signed the Emancipation Proclamation in 1863, putting an end to the horrible institution of slavery in our country, many slaves "tried" freedom but returned to their prior owners. Some never even ventured away from what they knew.

Why? Because slaves were dependent on their owners. They were afraid, and understandably so, that they could not make it on their own. President Lincoln could not change the slave mentality of an entire nation overnight. Neither could he reeducate former slaves and slave owners to give them the tools needed to work within this new paradigm.

At the risk, but certainly not the intention, of minimizing the plight of African Americans in our history, dieters face the same dynamic. We face our nation's diet mentality. We have been brainwashed to think we must depend on Weight Watchers, Bob Greene, Jenny Craig, exercising, eating healthy, etc. to lose weight. We are afraid to rely on our own choices. We have been shown over and over again if we do leave a program and are left to our own devices we will indeed gain the weight back and more.

Taking our choices back from our nation's diet mentality may sound simple at first, but you will be surprised at how frightening it can be. You should hear the fear and disbelief in the voice of a new client when I tell them we will be meeting at their favorite restaurant. They often stutter and stammer.

Their replies include things like, "But I haven't eaten there in years!" and "I can't be responsible for what I might eat there!" I have even detected tears on the other end of the phone line. And even after several exhilarating and successful consultations, if a client hits a little snag while implementing this new concept into their lives, they are so tempted to give up and run back to the industry with the 0.4% success rate!

So let me go into a little more detail why it's imperative you go through the process of taking off those diet shackles and taking your choices back.

Does Jenny Craig Really Know You?

There are over 300 million people living in our country and each one of us is living a distinctly different life. Each one of us is experiencing a multitude of different combinations of relationships, environments, and circumstances.

Think about how different we are – our body chemistries, our tastes in clothing, our ways of communicating, our family and cultural backgrounds, our experiences in 3rd grade, and the traumas and triumphs we've been through. Consider the myriad of different pieces of information we have stored in that data bank we call "our brain" and the different ways each of us interpret that information.

The variables are mind-boggling! And those variables are what influence our preferences and choices in life. Consciously or unconsciously, they affect every little decision we make during the day including what we feel like eating and doing at any particular time. Even the people who know us best probably couldn't predict what we are going to feel like eating tonight. You might not even be able to predict what you are going to want to eat for dinner tonight.

So wouldn't it be absolutely ridiculous to think that Jenny Craig, who is sitting in her multi-million dollar home in another part of the country, would know what you were craving for dinner? Would she know how much you were craving, and where you wanted to eat what you were craving? Does Jenny

Craig know what kind of day you had, or if you had time to eat lunch, or if it's that dreaded hormonal time of the month, or if the elevator was broken and you had to run up four flights of stairs to get to your office? Of course not!

But all these factors, consciously or unconsciously, will influence what you will be craving for dinner tonight. So why are you letting Jenny Craig choose the time, place, and menu? I'll tell you right now, she's not even going to show up for the date! And neither is Bob Greene, Suzanne Sommers, Dr. Phil, or any other of the diet and exercise gurus out there. And you're going to give up your choices to them?

" Tomorrow, Tomorrow, I Love Ya Tomorrow "

As previously discussed, when our choices are made for us, we become angry and resentful because it takes away our personal freedom, and inevitably there will be a backlash. Without question, all of my clients have experienced this backlash in one form or another, and it is the major reason for the weight to be regained and more.

This strong reaction comes in a devastating two-punch - physical as well as mental. Again nature is working against the dieter because it not only avoids deprivation, it prepares for it.

A dramatic example of this is the bear which can literally spend months in hibernation without eating. In anticipation of this, the bear's metabolism slows down dramatically and the bear is able to gain enormous amounts of weight right before and after the hibernation period. Studies show that our metabolism works similarly. If our body anticipates yet another diet, our metabolism will slow down much like the bear's.

But that particular factor doesn't even compare to the damage caused by the psychological part of this conundrum. It would be difficult for me to find a dieter who hasn't said at least one of the following on a great many occasion: "Oh, it's the weekend. I'll get back on my diet Monday morning," "I'm on vacation. When I get home I'll be good," "It's the holidays, I'm going to really get serious in the New Year," or "I've already blown it today, I'll start again tomorrow."

At first glance, these statements seem relatively harmless, even logical, but the psychological dynamic is more powerful than you can imagine. If you look at the statements above, every one of them has the surrender of choices as its accepted presumption to weight loss. There is no question presently the dieter feels he is exercising his real choices and later he will have to give them up. But even the dieter's real choices at this particular time are completely out of focus because of the psychological anticipation of giving them up.

In other words, when you use the words or a similar variation of the words, "I'll start tomorrow", it creates the dangerous psychological environment for eating way too much of your real choices because you anticipate not having them in the future.

Let me say that again because this very dynamic is one of the major factors that has contributed to our country's obesity problem. *When you use the words, 'I'll start tomorrow', it creates the dangerous psychological environment for eating way too much of your real choices because you anticipate not having them in the future.*

If you are a diet dropout, I would bet similar words have even crossed your mind while reading this book. Some readers have probably even smudged some of these pages with chocolate or orange residue from a bag of Cheetos thinking this might be their last chance to eat these forbidden foods before the New Rules are implemented.

Without question our brains are the most powerful source when it comes to the ultimate success or sabotage of losing weight. This is exactly why the New Rules works with your head rather than trying to fight against it. It is in our brain where psychological backlashes begin to create very physical reactions.

Your brain is capable of taking those seemingly harmless words, "I'll start tomorrow" and actually making your body *crave* enormous amounts of the food you will be giving up tomorrow. How many times have you said, "I don't know why I'm eating this, I'm not hungry"? Is it because somehow your brain knows of your intention to diet in the near future and you'll have to give it up?

From this point forward, if "I'll start tomorrow" or something similar to those words pass through your head in regards to starting a weight loss program, I want a huge red flag to be thrown in your brain! Without question you need to look at them as a warning signal tempting you back into the very unsuccessful weight loss world. You know through experience that those words have NEVER led you to permanent weight loss and they never will. You must remind yourself of that fact every time you hear them.

Don't Hate Me Because I'm a Donut

We've talked about one of the major psychological backlashes that lies at the bottom of our country's weight problem, and that is overeating in anticipation of having to give up our favorite foods. One of the others is caused by how the weight loss industry has made food a moral issue for us.

There is no better or more blatant example of this than the advertising cliché of the little angel and little devil sitting on a dieter's shoulder as he laments over what to eat. The devil tempts the dieter with a brownie deemed to be "bad" while the angel encourages the dieter to be "good" by eating a salad.

There are a million variations on this idea and they haven't been wasted on us. It has become so ingrained in our personal lexicons that we don't hesitate to refer to food as 'good' or 'bad' in our everyday vocabulary. And even more interesting and perhaps more telling is we commonly refer to ourselves as being 'bad' or 'good' when it comes to the food we eat.

Initially this may seem like a relatively harmless correlation, but let me reassure you our brains take it much more seriously. The words that stem from this correlation eventually lead to the other words like 'cheating', 'guilt', and 'failure'. By attaching these words to food, the weight loss industry has only created a more psychologically dangerous environment for our country which again has led us to overeat.

There are very few of us who haven't fallen off a diet by eating something 'bad' and then said, "Oh,

I've already blown it!" Then we proceed to polish off the entire bag of Oreos. Of course this leads us to feeling 'badly' about ourselves which causes us to eat more. It's a vicious and dangerous cycle which leads us to the diet hell of failing, binging, self-loathing, depression, and more overeating.

Additionally, it's not surprising to many of us if you put a 'forbidden' sign on anything, the attraction towards that particular thing immediately increases. Anyone who has ever been on a diet knows this is all the more true when we talk about forbidding a certain food. That food takes on a power that we wouldn't have even imagined before the diet!

All of this leads to an increasingly unhealthy relationship with food - overeating the 'bad' food when we 'fall off the wagon'.

The reality is food is not 'good' or 'bad'. A donut may not be as nutritional as a carrot but that doesn't make it 'bad', just less nutritional. An apple doesn't go to heaven while a brownie goes to hell. Respectively, the person eating them doesn't determine his eternal destination by what he chooses to eat. Nor does food define our moral integrity while we're here on earth. Think about how very ridiculous that notion is!

With the New Rules, not only is it imperative but it is required to stop referring to our food and ourselves as 'bad'. Now that you are aware of this dynamic, you will be surprised how many times a day you will hear people talking about their eating or themselves in terms of "good" and "bad". You will even catch yourself saying it many times without thinking. Again, I want a huge red flag to be thrown in your brain every time you hear it! It is this very mentality which has contributed to America's rise in eating disorders and obesity!

Remember that food is more or less nutritional and we may or may not choose to eat something more or less nutritional. That's it, period. Luckily we live in a time when vitamins are affordable and accessible to all of us. Studies show even those Americans who eat the healthiest diet don't get all the daily nutritional requirements from the food they eat and would benefit from a vitamin supplement.

Personally speaking, I choose less nutritional foods than the experts say I should be eating, but I can't remember the last time I was ill. Without hesitation, I attribute the latter to the vitamins I take on a daily basis. With or without the New Rules, everyone should be considering vitamin supplements.

McDonald's is in Our Genes

I happily and shamelessly admit right here I eat at McDonald's at least two or three times a week. McDonald's fries are one of the things I live for and oh, did I mention that I've been a size 4 for the last 15 years? My daughter, Brooke, who is presently 14, shares my passion for McDonald's and has since she had her first french fry at age 1 ½.

Although my daughter is surrounded by diet-obsessed classmates, she is happy, healthy and thin. Does she spend a lot of time in athletics? No. Just like her mother, PE is her least favorite class. If given a choice, she would much rather spend time talking on the phone than going on a bike ride.

So how has my daughter defied the odds? Is it in her genes? If it were, she and I would be headed towards the 200-pound weight which tends to run in my family. If Brooke inherited anything from me it was her love for McDonald's. Aside from that, the New Rules rule out the gene theory. Even though there is some evidence of genetics having a small percentage to do with predisposition towards obesity, I believe the chances are more likely parents pass down their unhealthy attitudes and obsessions about food rather than there being a physical link.

I know the idea of scientists finding a 'fat gene' is an awfully seductive idea to explain away our weight problem, but why would a 'fat gene' become such a problem in just the last 30 years? Where was it before? Evolutionary changes in human genetic codes happen over thousands and even tens of thousands of years, not thirty! And why would the obesity gene show up in epidemic proportions just here in America rather than other places in the world? It prefers the weather here? No, the New Rules will show you a much simpler explanation.

My daughter has had the benefit of growing up with a mother who knew there was something desperately wrong with the fact that even though America's obsessed with diet and exercise, Americans are getting fatter and fatter. Brooke has seldom doubted she can trust her own body and her own choices. She has an extremely healthy relationship with all of her favorite foods including McDonald's fries and chocolate shakes.

In that way, she will probably never need the rules because she is innately using them. I have never allowed her to buy into what the weight loss industry has everyone else buying into and what many of her young friends are buying into now. Whenever she brings up something she's heard on TV or read in a magazine about diet and exercise in regards to weight, I remind her she and I don't follow any of that advice and we're thinner than most of America.

There have been a few times during my daughter's lifetime she was worried about getting fat - an unfortunate byproduct of talking with her peers. Those times usually coincided with an increased appetite and a tighter fit of her favorite jeans. I would simply remind her that her body was just getting ready to go through a growth spurt. Without exception, a month later the tight waist line on her pants was loose again but the pant legs were an inch shorter.

Undoubtedly, one of the greatest casualties the weight loss industry has left in its wake is simple common sense. The New Rules help to infuse common sense back into our eating and into our lives.

As for my beloved favorite fast food restaurant, the weight loss industry has even managed to scare a little common sense out of them. McDonald's executives are seriously considering offering fresh fruit or cut vegetables as an option to their french fries in their children's Happy Meals! I can see it now – an epidemic of screaming children throwing themselves to the floors of McDonald's around the world!

France and Fat

It makes me crazy when I see weight loss experts push the notion, "Eat to live! Don't live to eat!" Bob Greene integrated it into Oprah's contract. The theory is we should consider food simply as fuel for our bodies, making our choices intellectually for the good of our body. The other part of the theory is we should take the emotion out of our food choices and we should, under no circumstances, use food to comfort ourselves. WHAT?!?! Everything about this theory simply defies common sense!

From the moment we are born, we associate food with comfort and emotion! Breast feeding is the epitome of correlating food with comfort and emotion! Eating is and was always meant to be a very sensual, pleasurable, nurturing, and satisfying experience. For anyone to suggest otherwise is nonsense.

Let's set aside the argument about less nutritional processed foods for a moment and just look at the colors and tastes which can be more directly attributed to our Creator. God made fruits and vegetables brightly colored and flavorful to insure people and animals would be attracted to them and eat them. Food is supposed to be appealing to our senses - it was how God made sure we wouldn't starve ourselves - *duh!* Of course that's not our problem anymore, but making us feel guilty about giving into what appeals to our senses, again sets us up for the backlash of overeating.

The alternative - giving into our senses, truly and completely enjoying any food we crave, and not feeling guilty about it - is the sure way to permanent weight loss. But don't just take my word for it, there's a whole country in Europe which proves this theory to be true.

You can disagree all you want with its politics, but France has the lowest obesity rate in all of Europe and puts America's statistics of obesity to shame. How is that possible when the French meal can often contain more fat than a meal at McDonald's? How is that possible when the streets of France are lined with shop windows full of beautifully butter-laden pastries?

How is that possible when the French unabashedly admit they love to linger over a good meal with good wine and good friends? How is that possible when the French pretty much break every rule America's weight loss industry has taught us?

These facts have so befuddled American scientists they have given it a published scientific title called The French Paradox. I was absolutely ecstatic when I found out about the French Paradox. It would have cost me literally millions of dollars and many, many years and many case studies to have gotten the scientific results needed to support the New Rules the way the French Paradox supports them. So what's the story?

The best way to examine what the French are doing is to first examine what they are generally not doing. The average Frenchman doesn't have any idea, or the interest for that matter, in how many calories, fat grams, or carbohydrates which are in the meals he is eating. He has no interest in how his food is combined or if it falls within *The Zone*. He rarely turns down the opportunity to celebrate or socialize with food and it would never occur to him to "exercise off" a meal after eating one.

When asked by an American doctor, Claude Fischler, a French sociologist and co-author of a French Paradox study explains what else the French don't do, "[American's] underlying notion is that food is dangerous and poisonous and you would be better off if you could avoid food all together……We don't have that. Food is OK."

What the French are doing is absolutely loving and savoring their cheeses, pastries, foie gras, and wine. And the thought of feeling guilty about doing so is a truly bazaar concept to the French. Fischler answers with his own question when asked about what would be most beneficial for Americans to take away from the study: "Can we figure out how to rid the Americans of their guilt and their concern and their anxiety toward food?"

One of the wonderful benefits of the French's absence of guilt, anxiety, and even their lack of interest in the nutritional content of their food is they do not deal with the same psychological backlashes that Americans constantly deal with. The French don't overeat in anticipation of not being able to eat their favorite foods in the future. The French don't feel "badly" about themselves when they eat a pastry. They don't overeat because they have a healthy relationship with food.

We talked briefly about how fat is one of the physical factors of satiety. The French diet certainly contains fat and interestingly enough, primarily the fat that American scientists have deemed 'bad' fat.

The French, however, only use the word 'bad' in regards to food when something doesn't taste good. When something ***does*** taste good it fulfills a huge part of the satiety equation - what pleases our senses of sight, smell, and taste.

As discussed before, those things that please our senses at any particular time can be as individual as we are, so the French would never think to let someone else decide that for them. The French eat what looks good, smells good, and tastes good to them at the time. They know they will do this for their next meal, and their next, and their next until their last day.

There is no desperate overeating because they have 'fallen off the wagon' – the French never get in the wagon! I can just imagine a Frenchman holding a glass of wine and saying with his French accent, "Why get in a wagin wiz no weels? It is not zat exciting. Za scenary – it duz not shange."

Scientists know our emotions and thoughts are capable of affecting the chemicals our bodies excrete into our bloodstream. That would be no less true in relation to the guilt-free pleasure or the painful anxiety we experience while eating. Those chemicals can respectively be beneficial or detrimental to our health.

We've all heard about the stories of terminally ill patients literally curing their illnesses with positive self-talk and visualization. When applied to the French Paradox, scientists are considering the chemicals the French body might excrete may be beneficial while the American body may excrete detrimental chemicals even when eating the same meal. Those chemicals may even override any healthy or unhealthy affects the actual food ingested would incur in the body.

Whatever the reasons and the science behind the French Paradox, another product of having the healthy relationship with food the French have with food is there are very few if any all-you-can-eat buffets in France. In the next chapter you will see, for Americans, it is a much bigger issue in more ways than one.

Getting Your Money's Worth

All You Can Eat for $3.99!!! Super Size Your Meal for 39¢! You don't live in America if you've never seen ads like that before! I'm not sure if this culture of Bigger-is-Better started way back when we first colonized this very big piece of land we call the United States, but there is no denying Americans are capitalistically minded. We are generally interested in getting as much as we can for our dollar and I'm no different.

It is unfortunate the weight loss industry has dismissed this marketing ploy of getting more for our money and instead blames the actual food content for our obesity. But one of the major factors for our bigger bodies is our belief that we are getting such a good deal when we can buy (and eat) 2 cheeseburgers for the price of one.

There are a lot of headlines lately involving certain fast food companies and their overweight customers. Customers are actually suing these companies, trying to make them responsible for their own obesity problems. This is ABSURD! The only thing these companies are responsible for is tapping into the getting-your-money's-worth mentality to sell more of their product. This sales approach isn't anything new and all sound retail businesses utilize it.

Like most people, I love the idea of getting a good deal, but I know when it comes to food, all-you-can-eat buffets and supersized meals are a complete waste of money. Let me explain why.

Let's say you go ahead and go to the all-you-can-eat buffet at Pizza Hut. You eat 6 pieces of pizza,

2 servings of pasta salad, 2 pieces of lasagna, 1 green salad, and 2 servings of ice cream for dessert, all for $3.99! Now, let's say you and your body only needed and would have been perfectly satisfied with 2 pieces of pizza, 1 serving of pasta, 1 green salad, and the ice cream.

That means all the rest – let's estimate an extra 3500 calories – is going to go into your body where you are either going to have to pay Jenny Craig or some other program $10, $20, $30 or more to help you get it off your body. That buffet lunch could cost you upwards of $33.99 or more! But let's not forget those programs have been proven unsuccessful when helping you lose the weight for good. You could feasibly spend 3, 4, or 5 times that amount to get off the 3500 calories which was such a good deal at the all-you-can-eat buffet!

You might be thinking you would never overeat 3500 calories in a single meal, but this equation applies to every single bite of food your body is not going to use at any meal. Let's say you order what you would consider an ordinary size American meal – I make the American distinction because in the countries which have not yet tapped into the American Bigger-is-Better mentality, the meal sizes are, poignantly enough, significantly smaller.

Anyway, you go ahead and finish the whole cheeseburger, all the fries, and the last sip of the chocolate shake. Now let's say you and your body would have been perfectly satisfied had you left 3 bites of your burger, 7 french fries, and 5 sips of your chocolate shake, but you didn't want to waste that food.

Let's give those bites you could have left on your plate an approximate 200 calorie value and 95¢

monetary value. Because you did not want to waste 95¢, the 200 calories your body didn't need will now go into being fat on your body. It would only take about a week of eating those extra bites and you would have gained one pound. Again you will have to spend much more money to get the weight off your body than it would have cost if you would have just left those bites on your plate.

Let's consider what else eating all that 'good deal' food cost you. One of the wonderful things about this body we have is how the organ of our stomach works. It is physically capable of expanding and retracting; a mechanism that was meant to help us adjust to periods of deprivation and plenty in ages gone by. However, now we live in a time when our stomachs rarely need to retract because of the accessibility and abundance of food.

What is so unfortunate about this scenario is Americans have been using the feeling of stomach fullness as their primary feeling of satiety (point of satisfaction). Remember the weight loss industry has essentially taken away our most powerful satiety factor - eating and fully enjoying the foods which we crave, love, and want to eat at any particular time without feeling guilty.

We've been told instead the feeling of our stomachs being full is when we're really satisfied. There are plenty of books perpetuating this idea and just making things worse in the long run. The book, *Eat More, Weigh Less* says it blatantly in its title. The whole idea is to allow a dieter to physically fill up the stomach with 'legal' or 'free' foods so he won't feel hungry.

Another popular version of this form of dieting shows you a small piece of 'bad' food like a piece of cheesecake and then shows you some bulkier 'good' foods like a half a melon, a couple of graham crackers, and a bowl of fat-free air-popped popcorn. All of the latter you can eat instead of the small cheesecake.

Well, have you tried it? Of course you have! And it doesn't work long term, does it? Of course it doesn't because filling up the stomach is actually one of the least powerful factors for true satisfaction. In fact, now all we've done is physically stretched out our stomachs because we think we have to feel 'stuffed' to be satisfied.

Then to make matters worse, when we inevitably 'fall off the wagon' we go to the all-you-can-eat buffet and stuff our newly stretched out stomachs with what the weight loss industry has deemed 'bad' food. It's a safe bet the 'bad food' has many more calories per square inch than the bushel full of vegetables we had been eating on the diet! Is it any wonder we are fatter than ever?!?!

Lastly, the financial consequences of any medical problems brought on by eating more than your body needs is almost immeasurable and should erase any doubt that supersized meals and all-you-can-eat buffets are incredibly expensive in the long run. As a general rule of thumb, don't bother with them.

Children and The Clean Plate Club

You may not be one of the all-you-can-eat buffet eaters mentioned in the previous chapter, but there's a good possibility that you grew up in a home which had a version of The Clean Plate Club. Unfortunately, very few of us got out of our childhood without some skewed thoughts about food. If they go unrecognized, these are the same ones you are bound to pass on to the children in your life.

How many of us remember our parents saying "Clean your plate. There are children in Africa that are starving!" Think about how psychologically unsound that premise is! Our parents were encouraging us to overeat by making us feel guilty! Even though few of us would say what we were really thinking for fear of punishment, we wanted to tell our parents, "Well, then send them the rest of the food on my plate!" Although that may sound defiant and disrespectful to most parents, it is ultimately a much more psychologically healthy statement.

Children are born with an innately healthy relationship with food. I'm not saying left unmonitored, children wouldn't choose to eat less healthy foods, but they are much more in touch with their hunger and satiety signals - that is, until adults get in there and start messing things up.

Aside from the example above, there was also the psychologically unsound scenario of holding the dessert hostage until you ate everything on your plate. Remember that? We had to overeat to be 'good' in order to have the dessert. So early on, we associated a clean plate to being "good" and "guilt-free" - very powerful messages that we take into our adulthood.

I can't tell you how hard it is for some of my clients to leave food on their plates and how uncomfortable it makes them feel. It is because they feel the deep seeded guilt their parents instilled in them as a child. Those same clients feel overwhelming guilt when they have overeaten. It is a no-win situation. Additionally, we learned early to give dessert a much higher and desirable place in our relationship to food because our parents made it a reward instead of just another course in the meal.

From the time my daughter was very young, her father and I disagreed on this issue. Brooke's father grew up, as most of us, with a membership to the clean plate club with the hostage dessert addendum. He would have liked to see his daughter follow suit to some extent. What makes this a little more surprising is his distinct memory of throwing up the peas his father insisted he finish off his plate.

However, Brooke's father did travel the majority of the time so by default she was subject to my philosophy regarding eating. I, of course, encouraged healthy choices with Brooke, but I didn't treat the less healthy choices too much differently. She could eat until she was satisfied, leave the rest, and still have dessert. The amazing thing, or maybe not so amazing, is that oftentimes she would leave much of the dessert as well.

As a result, Brooke presently doesn't feel real strongly about any food and can make healthier choices without too much struggle. Of course, she knows she can always have ice cream whenever she wants also. And even more importantly, she never fell out of touch with her natural signals of hunger and satiety which is why she is not overweight.

Unfortunately, as the statistics show, more and more children are overweight today and there is also a significant rise in eating disorders amongst children. Too many parents today not only pass down their own childhood issues with food but all the additional diet mentality messages they've collected in the last 30 years. Do kids even have a chance?

When I watch programs about obesity and children, the interviews are heartbreaking. Children as young as 4 or 5 refer to foods as "bad" and say they mustn't eat them any more. Their vocabulary also includes words like "cheating" and "failing".

I've seen children as young as 14 who have lost and regained hundreds of pounds since they were six, but have never been able to keep the weight off. Many have been to "fat camps" where they are only destined to be more programmed with the erroneous messages we have talked about in other chapters in this book. They return to their parents several pounds thinner, but spend the rest of the year regaining it back and more. To make matters increasingly worse, parents become "food police" continually nagging these children and making them feel badly for what they "should" or "shouldn't" be eating.

It is difficult enough for adults to deal with the diet messages we get from the media and the nagging we get from other adults. Can you imagine being a child and having the most important people in your life making you feel guilty and badly about eating on a daily basis?! It is absolutely maddening for me to see what these parents are unknowingly doing to their children!!

Those children being interviewed sit there bloated, hopeless, and helpless. More alarmingly, they continue to be in grave danger of even more backlash overeating. Doesn't anyone see they are suffering even more from the mentality of the weight loss industry because their parents are now the very personification of that industry?

So not only is it important to turn in your Clean Plate membership cards and learn these New Rules, but we must insist our children do the same. And the importance of being able to leave food on your plate and encouraging your children to leave food on their plate cannot be stressed enough. This is explained in more detail in the chapter, *The New Rules are Born,* but first let's demystify why America is really overweight.

The Simple Equation (This One's for You, Dr. Phil)

64.5% of Americans are not overweight because of fast food and lack of activity. They are overweight because they are consuming more calories than they are expending. When you eat more calories than you expend, you gain weight. If you eat fewer calories than you expend, you lose weight. That's it. That's the simple equation.

From the standpoint of weight gain and loss, it doesn't matter much if those calories come from your favorite foods or a head of lettuce. It doesn't matter much if you're training for a marathon or sitting at a desk all day. If you eat more calories than you burn, you will gain weight. If you eat less than you expend, you will lose weight.

The approximate 25% of adults who can be considered obese are obese because they have consumed an obese number of calories over and above what they expended. How many times have you seen an obese person interviewed on TV, saying obesity runs in their family? Then inevitably we find out they are eating ridiculous amounts of food like a dozen eggs and a loaf of bread for breakfast alone?!

If people are overeating, they have an unhealthy relationship with food. The more food a person is overeating is directly in proportion to the unhealthiness of their relationship to food, not their relationship to unhealthy foods.

Carnie Wilson, the singer-daughter of the late Mama Cass who herself was obese, had a terrible problem with her weight. She weighed over 300 pounds when she decided to undergo a very serious surgical procedure that reduced the size of her stomach to the size of a quarter. Should it surprise us that she lost over 150 pounds in less than 15 months? She couldn't eat more than a few bites before she was nauseatingly full!

The completely astonishing thing about Wilson's story though is she appears to still have a very unhealthy relationship with food. I read in an interview recently she rarely eats bread because she feels guilty if she does!

The fact is if your stomach is the size of a quarter, you can eat bread all day, every day for the rest of your life and still lose weight because you would be eating very little bread! You would not be getting as much nutrition as Wilson gets by sticking to the "healthy" diet that her doctors have her on, but Wilson hardly gets any nutrition from the food she eats anyway because of how little she eats.

Admittedly, Wilson has to take a good deal of vitamins to supplement her diet. As previously discussed, studies show even Americans who eat the healthiest of diets with bigger portions, still don't get all the nutrition they need from the foods they eat. Taking vitamins is sound advice for anyone regardless of the kind of food or the amount of food you consume.

Wilson was also put on an exercise regimen by her doctors but one that ensued only after she had had time to recover from her surgery. But even before her exercise regimen started, Wilson had already lost a significant amount of weight, and she would have continued to lose weight with or without the added exercise.

Again, not to say exercise is not a healthy thing to do. We all know what exercise can do to strengthen and tone our bodies and burn calories, but the fact is you **do not** have to exercise to lose weight. Certainly not to minimize a horrendous time in history, but rather to make a powerful point: There were no gyms at Auchwitz.

What you do need to do to lose weight, whether you spend all day in bed watching TV or whether you teach aerobics 8 hours a day, is take in less than you expend. This simple equation is the common sense which makes up the basis for the New Rules.

And guess what else? Your body was built to know what your activity level is at any particular time and how many calories it needs to sustain that activity. The weight loss industry has turned that upside down, making us think we have to consciously choose activity to expend the calories we've already overeaten.

Your body is even capable of shrinking your stomach on its own without major surgery. The human body will always know more about the science of weight loss than the scientists will know. Unfortunately, we can thank the weight loss industry for not allowing our bodies do what they were meant to do.

People like Bob Greene and Dr. Phil, although well intended, have joined the rest of the weight loss industry by making weight loss an incredibly complicated and difficult issue. Unfortunately, the more difficult they make it, the much more likely a dieter will "fail" and, in turn, overeat.

In his book, *The Ultimate Weight Solution,* Dr. Phil boldly claims he has decoded America's reasons for being overweight and his way is the only real way to lose weight permanently.

Aside from the obvious criticism that Dr. Phil himself is not very svelte, his solution is a metaphorical Mount Everest to climb. He lays out a laborious program which starts with intensive self-therapy, throwing out all your favorite foods, and committing to exercising. Then he asks you to rid your life of any friends, family, or even career choices which would cause you to eat "bad" food! And he has the gall to say his program has nothing to do with dieting or willpower?! COME ON! HE'S KIDDING, RIGHT?

All Dr. Phil has done is create an even more dangerous environment for his readers and viewers for backlash overeating. No doubt, he will find a thousand or so success stories at the end of the year to display on his television program who bought into giving *him* the power to lose *their* weight, but how about the other 2,499,952 people who read his book and failed? They'll be overeating and gaining even more weight! And the odds of the 1000 success stories staying successfully thin over a significant period of time is equally as bleak.

Rather than forcing Americans to have a healthy lifestyle and eat healthy foods, Americans first need to have a healthy relationship with whatever lifestyle they choose and whatever food they choose to eat. If Americans had a healthy relationship with food, for the most part it wouldn't matter what they were eating or how much they were exercising. They would consume what their particular body needed on any particular day.

Our bodies were built to know the difference in activity. If couch potatoes were in tune to their bodies, they could still be thin eating their favorite fast food but they would be eating much less of it. And because those couch potatoes wouldn't feel overwhelmed and guilty every time they ate something, they would even be more apt to make healthier choices on other occasions.

The New Rules are Born

As discussed in the chapter, *Children and The Clean Plate Club*, being able to leave food on your plate is very important in implementing the New Rules. What became the seed for the New Rules was a simple segment I watched on a morning show. There was a nutritionist who stood in front of a table overloaded with food, and the nutritionist said, "If you were to leave a few bites of food on your plate every meal for a year, this is the amount of food you would **not** be eating. This equals about 20 lbs. which you would not put on your body."

I do believe an actual light bulb appeared over my head at that very moment! After all the years of desperate dieting, I knew the one thing I could do is leave a few bites of food on my plate! So that very afternoon, I went to my favorite restaurant and ordered my favorite food. But for the first time I left a few bites of the sandwich, a few bites of french fries, about a quarter of the chocolate chip milkshake and about 6 bites of the apple pie ala mode.

Looking back, it's hard to imagine I was eating such a large quantity of food. But my relationship with food was so out of whack at that point, I had built up a hefty consumption.

Initially it was a little difficult to leave the food on the plate. I did not like the idea of "wasting" food but I kept thinking, 'I'd rather waste it on the plate than waste it on my waist.' So while waiting for the waitress to come get the plate, I took the salt shaker and poured salt all over the remaining food and in the shake so I wouldn't pick at it.

Once that salt was poured, something incredible happened. My whole paradigm changed. Seeing and knowing I could leave food on my plate and knowing it was not going to turn into fat on my body gave me such a sense of power over it. I had suffered so long under the power of food thanks to the diet industry. It felt like the weight of the world had tumbled off my shoulders. Little did I know the weight on my hips would soon follow!

I felt as if I literally jumped off the merry-go-round and I couldn't believe how easy it was! I could have whatever I wanted to eat from then on as long as I could leave a little on my plate. And at the end of that first day, I went to bed thinking about all the food I ***didn't*** eat instead of agonizing about all the food I did eat as I had so many nights before. It truly felt like the shackles had been taken off my wrists and ankles! 'And tomorrow morning,' I thought as I fell asleep peacefully that night, 'I get to have French toast!'

As days and weeks went by, a few bites turned into a lot more bites left on my plate. The only little decision I had to make during any meal was when I would use the salt shaker. The fact I no longer had to deny myself and ate only what I really craved had put me back in touch with my true satiety point. I was satisfying the most powerful factor when it comes to our relationship with food - my head - all that data which influenced my food choices for whatever emotional, physical, or mental reason. And in so doing, it took less and less food to satisfy me. It brought me back to being in touch with my body and even more importantly, it took all the fear out of eating.

This is the very point which is so important to

make and is being dealt with erroneously by today's so-called weight loss experts - ***we have a strong emotional connection to food. That connection should be honored, not denied!***

In a healthy relationship with food, you can have comfort food comfort you if you've had a bad day. It's similar to a healthy relationship with your partner - he or she is supposed to be there for comfort when you need comforting. However, something's definitely unhealthy with a relationship if you need constant and incessant comforting. In our relationships with people, if we think they may not be there in the future, we can't get enough of their comfort. The psychological backlash of anticipating the loss of your favorite foods is the same.

Feeling powerful and in control around any food and having the freedom to eat anything you desire at any particular time is the very basis of a healthy relationship with food. The New Rules are designed to get you back to that place.

What happened to me and what is ultimately the goal of the New Rules could be likened to putting someone in a beautiful dining room with a buffet full of their favorite foods constantly at hand and fresh to the taste. With the absolute assurance of losing 10 pounds no matter what or how much was eaten, we would keep that person there for a full month.

What do you think would happen at the end of the 30 days? That person would come out of that room with a healthy relationship with food! Food would no longer hold the power or significance it did while dieting. It would simply be food, delicious, yes – to be enjoyed, absolutely – to be chosen when wanted, yes– but never to be a slave to again.

And on the last day of the time in the "buffet room" I guarantee that person would be eating significantly less food than he did on the first day. Food, just like anything in life, gets much less appealing when you truly know you can have it whenever you want and without consequences.

The New Rules are designed to put food back into the proper context in your life. But since the aforementioned scenario is obviously unrealistic, we'll be doing it one little delicious bite at a time!

Jogging on a Dinner Plate

In the chapter, *Getting Your Money's Worth,* we talked about giving bites of food left on your plate a caloric and monetary value to demonstrate the ridiculousness of the all-you-can-eat buffet. For the purpose of showing you the powerful yet simple physical implications of leaving food on your plate, the New Rules give every bite of food left on your plate an average value of 25 calories. Some foods obviously will have less calories in a bite and some more. But since the New Rules will be allowing all foods and *not* allowing obsession with calorie counting, we've given it a simple average.

Let's say, as we did similarly before, you leave 4 bites of a sandwich, 2 bites of french fries, and 3 bites of pie on your plate this afternoon at lunch when you ordinarily would have eaten everything. That would be 9 bites of food which you did ***not*** eat. 9 x 25 = 225. This means you did ***not*** put 225 calories in your body you will have to burn off.

Now consider the fact it would take a mile of jogging to burn about 100 calories. Because you left 9 bites of food on your plate you ***will not*** have to jog 2 ¼ miles! Which is easier, leaving 9 bites of food on your plate or jogging 2 ¼ miles? In short, every bite of food that you do not eat is a quarter mile you do not have to jog! We call this *jogging on a dinner plate.*

So when you're tempted to grab back your clean plate club membership card, visualize a waste bin with one of those post office box openings swung open and then your belly with the same opening. Then ask yourself which one are you going to scrape your leftovers into?

It is better to waste on your plate, then waste on your waist! And it is so much easier to go jogging on a dinner plate then mustering up the motivation to actually strap on the jogging shoes and sweating for an hour or two every day! Would you agree?

To Exercise or Not to Exercise: That is the Question

So what about really exercising? To reiterate for the umpteenth time, ideally, all of us should be on an exercise regimen for the healthful benefits. Unfortunately, that's just not going to happen. Generally speaking, people don't like to exercise and they don't want to exercise. Fortunately, it is not necessary to lose weight.

If you haven't already noticed, this book wasn't meant to be politically correct when it comes to the issues of healthy eating and exercise. It was meant to be realistic about why those things aren't working when it comes to losing weight permanently. As stated before, you simply need to consume less than you expend to lose weight.

Remember also that America's weight loss industry has caused us to put exercise in the erroneous context of having to exercise *after* we've eaten too much. That is like putting the cart before the horse. Our bodies were built to know how much we need to match our present activity level, not to have to consciously exercise off food we've already eaten.

What I will say is that if you hate to exercise as much as I do but recognize the benefits, you may want to incorporate it in a way that I have - by not complaining. I have stopped complaining about not finding a close parking spot at the grocery store or mall. I have stopped complaining about living on the third floor of our apartment building which has no elevator. I no longer complain about carrying six bags of groceries up those stairs when I have no one to help.

I try to vacuum twice a week. I'll be more apt to respond to the 'Take me for a walk' look on the face of our dogs. In other words, I look at the ordinarily tedious activity in my everyday life now in a different light. Not only does it keep me healthier physically, I no longer feel resentful for having to do it so my attitude is healthier as well.

A little note: On those rare occasions I do lift a 10-lb barbell and do some curls, it is extremely satisfying to see my muscles so easily since my arms are already thin but still not rewarding enough to be consistent. Go figure.

However, if you do want to do the more traditional exercising please don't waste your money on the latest infomercial exercise gadget. I and many of my friends and family have bought at least one of those machines and they all ended up in the same place. You know that place - either under the bed or in a garage sale! One day my husband and I even saw a perfectly good stair stepper dumped in our apartment garbage bin! Do you know why? Because you actually have to *use* the machine for it to work!

As discussed in the chapter, *Emancipating the Diet Slaves,* there's a reason why we have a natural aversion to exercise. It's the same reason those infomercials have to be so persuasively produced. They have you thinking if the machine is just sitting in your bedroom, your body will be magnetically and uncontrollably drawn to it and start exercising. But that doesn't happen for the same reason your carpet doesn't compel your body to get down on it and do push-ups and sit-ups.

To exercise or not exercise is up to you, but if you do decide on exercising make certain it is for the health benefits not losing weight. If you find yourself thinking, 'Well, I can eat more today because I exercised,' you're in dangerous diet mentality territory.

Many a client will tell me that they want to continue to exercise for the healthful benefits. I'm always suspicious when I hear that comment so I give them a litmus test of sorts by asking, "If I told you if you continued to exercise and would reap all the healthful benefits of exercising except it would keep you from losing any weight, would you continue to exercise?"

If the answer is no, then they haven't disconnected exercise with losing weight. And disconnecting the two is imperative to losing the diet mentality. The truth is you do not have to exercise to lose weight. If you attach exercise to losing weight you replace your natural body signals of eating according to your activity. Instead, you are telling your body you have to experience pain and effort to accomplish what your body should be doing naturally. The result will be rebellion and backlash in overeating.

You may want to wait until the rules have really been incorporated into your thinking and until you've already lost a good deal of weight before incorporating an exercise regimen. And again, do it for the health benefits not for the purpose of losing weight. Have I told you enough times how important it is to disassociate exercise with weight loss?

Regardless, you should always check with your physician before starting any exercise regimen. Oh, and use the carpet – it's a lot cheaper.

Changing Scales

Before we embark on the simple step-by-step rules in Part II of this book there are just a couple more things to discuss. One of those things is that little appliance which usually can be found sitting on your bathroom floor. What is not up for discussion is unequivocally, without question, it must go. Don't even bother reading Part II if you are not planning to get rid of all the scales in your home. THIS IS A NON-NEGOTIABLE POINT. Weigh yourself one last time if you must, but then throw it in the lake, donate it to the thrift store, or better yet, give it to someone you don't like.

If your partner or your family puts up a fuss, tell them they can weigh themselves at school, at the gym, at the neighbor's, or even at the grocery store for that matter, but there will no longer be any weighing of anything or anyone at home. From here on out and until you are wearing the size clothes you want to be wearing, you will not be stepping on a scale. If you must get weighed at your doctor's office, turn around and kindly ask the nurse to record it without announcing it verbally to you.

Why the big deal? Because along with giving so much power away to diet and exercise programs, we have given an incredible amount of power to that little thing with all those numbers. We've allowed scales to tell us if we've been "bad" or "good".

Scales also let you know if you've done enough or need to do more. Scales tell you how slowly or how quickly. Scales disapprove and disappoint. Dieters don't just allow scales to measure their weight, they allow scales to measure their self-worth.

How many times have you allowed your scale to completely determine what kind of day you're going to have? For all the same psychological backlash reasons that lead to overeating, the scale is undeniably one of your worst enemies when trying to lose weight, so get rid of it! NOW!! Don't go on reading. Get up and get rid of the scales and then come back and continue on with this chapter.......don't worry I'll wait....go on..............

Good. If it makes you feel any better I'm going to give you a new scale and it works so much better than the one you just threw out. It is called the Pleasure Scale. It's a simple scale from 1 - 10, 10 being the most pleasurable.

You will be using it to help you decide when you want to eat, what you want to eat, and when you're going to stop eating. The Pleasure Scale is in your head, so it doesn't cost you a thing. You can take it conveniently wherever you go, and it will be the key to getting back in touch with your own choices and restoring your relationship with food.

Remember the New Rules will not be doing what the diet industry has been trying to do - forcing you to have a relationship with healthy foods. The New Rules will be giving you back a healthy relationship to all foods.

Last Notes

As you well know by now, the New Rules are rather unorthodox when it comes to what we've been told by America's weight loss industry. So as you embark on this new way to weight loss, expect even the closest people to you to challenge this new thinking. Remember they have been just as brainwashed as the rest of us. You might even want to consider not sharing it with them until they notice your weight loss.

Stay very aware of the messages people will continue to send you which come straight from the very unsuccessful weight loss industry. Those would include, "I can't believe you're eating that when you're trying to lose weight!" or "You're never going to lose weight if you keep eating that "bad" food. You need to start exercising and eating right."

Beware of the friends who have lost weight on the latest fad diet! You have been there before! They've been there before! Continue on your new road and watch as their weight creeps back up and yours continues to go down.

If you have someone close who is really giving you a hard time, insist they read this entire book (not just glance through it). Then ask them to respectfully not say another word to you about it.

While you are learning to use the New Rules, be good to yourself. Go ahead and buy some new clothes now and look the best you can look all during this process. Don't fall into the diet mentality of, "When I lose all the weight, I'll buy a new wardrobe." And don't fall into the ridiculous theory of wearing tight clothes to remind you to stop eating! The only thing that screams to a diet dropout is "YOU NEED TO DIET!!!"

This new way of thinking not only includes enjoying food again right now but just enjoying being alive again, right now. If you're genuinely concerned about the financial implications of buying new clothes at this size and will eventually have to buy another set of clothes later, buy things you know you will be able to wear even when they get baggier like drawstring pants or slip dresses. You can be creative!

Additionally, you might have noticed there has been no mention of "time" when referring to the New Rules. The diet mentality is all about time. "Lose 5 lbs. in 3 days!" "Lose 10lbs in Time for Bikini Season!" "I want to lose 20 lbs before my wedding." If I could make you throw out time like I made you throw out your scale, I would.

It's not about the time. It's about losing weight permanently and getting to the point where you will never have to think twice about trying to lose weight before an upcoming event again. It's about eventually being thin all the time and looking forward to the food and fun that awaits you every day.

If there is an event coming up soon and you want to lose a certain amount of weight before the event, the diet mentality is speaking. Instead, I encourage you to find something special to wear which makes you feel great now and use the New Rules to really look forward to enjoying the food and drinks at the event.

I will give you a little bit of a break here by saying that my weight came off more quickly than I anticipated, but that is truly because I had given up on dieting and had little expectation. As long as I was getting smaller and still not feeling at all like I was depriving myself, it was easier and easier to leave more and more food on my plate.

Keeping that in mind, it's easy to see why the last half of the pounds I wanted to lose went the fastest. Again, this is in complete opposition to what the weight loss industry has taught us. How many times have we been told the last 10 pounds are the hardest?

Depending on how much food you are consuming, the first phase may be just slowing down the pace of weight gain. The second phase might be stopping the weight gain. The third phase would be slowly losing and the fourth would be quickly losing.

I was listening to a talk radio show the other day and a truck driver called into the show to share his weight loss story. A year and a half earlier he had been close to 400 pounds and now he was 210 pounds. At 6'3" and 69 years old, he was pretty proud of his weight loss.

The hosts were chomping at the bit to find out how he managed to exercise and eat right while he was on the road. He said he really didn't exercise at all, but he did start cutting down on his food. The truck driver went on to explain how he would throw away half his sandwiches and cut down on his snack stops. In the first couple of months, he didn't lose any weight, but then it just started to peel off!

The hosts were incredulous and almost rude! They even accused him of being a prank caller! People are so convinced losing weight has to be a disciplined and difficult task! This is simply not true and as long as people perpetuate that idea, we will only get heavier.

Unlike the truck driver, some diet dropouts will go directly to losing weight, but others might not. That is exactly why you have to get rid of your scale - because it could be devastating if it told you that you were not losing weight as quickly as you anticipated. Then no snack in the house will be safe!

IMPORTANT NOTE: You will probably lose more weight towards the end of your weight loss journey with the New Rules rather than the beginning. Regardless, never forget the simple fact what you don't put into your body will not have to be dieted or exercised off. Better waste on the plate than waste on your waist - it's much easier to jog on a dinner plate!

Lastly, relax. Most weight loss programs have the "white knuckling" effect built into them – bracing yourself for pain and deprivation. These New Rules were designed to keep the color in your knuckles. They are not going to punish you if you get off track at times. If you find yourself overeating at one time or another (*which you will*) or your pants are a little tighter than the day before (*Could it be that time of month?*), don't panic!

It doesn't mean you've failed or the New Rules failed. Just like learning how to drive on the right side of the road - you're not going to quit driving if you occasionally swerve into the left lane!

It is especially important at those times you go right back to enjoying your very next meal and applying the rules again. All the while you have to continue to remind yourself of the 0.4% success rates of any other diet options. The New Rules, I promise you, is the right side of the road and driving doesn't get any easier than this!

PART II

The New Rules for Diet Dropouts

Rule #1: Read Part I of This Book.

Don't skip right to the New Rules. I made a conscious effort to make this book a quick read and not bog it down full of facts and figures. My intention was to make it easy to read it over and over again in an effort to "rebrainwash" yourself.

It is imperative you know how and why these New Rules work and why everything else hasn't worked for you or the rest of America. And you need to remind yourself constantly of those very things.

You will be tempted more than you realize to rush back to the old way of thinking which the weight loss industry has instilled in all of us. But never forget it is a business with a less than 1% success rate for permanent weight loss!

Rule #2: Throw Away Your Scale!

If you did read Part I, you have already gotten rid of all the scales in your home. If you didn't read Part I, refer to Rule #1. If you've decided not to rid yourself of them, don't even bother reading on. It is one of the few rules with no room for negotiation.

You may weigh yourself one more time before throwing out your scales, but you must not weigh yourself again until you are wearing the size clothes you want to be wearing. And even then, it would be wise to never get on a scale again.

I can't remember the last time I weighed myself because even now, after 15 years of being a size 4, I realize what power that scale can wield in my life. It is, for reasons explained in the chapter *Changing Scales*, one of the worst enemies a person has in their journey to lose weight and maintaining that weight loss.

Rule #3: Take Your Vitamins and Drink Your Water

As discussed in Part I, recent studies have shown that every American would benefit from taking a daily multivitamin. I personally have a vitamin regimen including a multivitamin for women, an extra vitamin C, a fish oil capsule, extra B vitamins, and a soy supplement. I absolutely believe my faithful consumption of these can be credited for my continued health in spite of my food choices.

You should take some time to talk to your local vitamin store clerk, your doctor, or do some studying on your own about vitamins. Be aware certain vitamins can be toxic if taken in the wrong amounts, so be educated with your choices. Whatever your choice, MAKE SURE YOU DO CHOOSE! Especially while learning the New Rules, you should expect your food choices will lean towards less healthy choices, so vitamins are particularly important and will pick up the slack.

Even though we didn't touch on this subject before this time, do make sure you drink your water as well, preferably up to the recommended 8 glasses a day. I don't think I have to go into the benefits of drinking water. We have all heard them, and the New Rules support them, so DRINK!

Rule #4: Fill Out, Sign, and Date This Permission Slip

I, Susanna Wermuth, former dieter and former comrade in your misery in the quest to lose weight, give you, (*your name*) ____________________ ____________________, from this day, (*enter today's date*) ____________________ forward, the permission to eat anything you choose, anytime you choose, and still lose weight. I give you permission to really love food again and put it back into the proper perspective in your life so you can look forward to going out with friends, going on vacations, and eating at your favorite restaurants. I give you all your power and choices back from the media, people, and diet experts you have listened to and failed you in the past. I give you the permission to use these New Rules and enjoy this new road to permanent weight loss.

Signed: Susanna H. Wermuth

Agreed: (*your signature*) ____________________

Date: ____________________

Rule #5: Always Start Now!

The New Rules are always meant to be implemented in this very moment, right now. They are not something you will start tomorrow, next Monday, or after the holidays. There will be moments of relapse in overeating when using the New Rules. There will be days that your clothes will fit a little tighter than they did the day before.

Those are the very moments that you must make a conscious effort not to panic! Do not run back to the pathetically unsuccessful world of the weight loss industry. Instead, you must think about enjoying your next meal. Even after 15 years, I still have moments I momentarily panic and I have to remind myself of these very same things.

As mentioned before, while you are learning to drive on the right side of the road, you don't quit just because you swerve into the left lane occasionally. Even after you become an adept driver, you will occasionally be distracted and swerve a bit.

Rule #6: Relax

I know looking at and feeling the unwanted fat on your body can be a source of great anxiety and can make you feel hopeless and desperate. You want the fat to just be gone! Well, guess what? That's not going to happen. If there was a magic pill, America wouldn't have the obesity problem it presently has and a problem that continues to grow.

However, feeling hopeless and desperate can lead to a major binge. So do your best to take a deep breath and relax when those anxious feelings come your way. Then think about the next meal or snack you are going to enjoy!

Rule #7: Choose When to Eat with Your Pleasure Scale

Whenever you think about eating, first remind yourself no one is ever going to make you give up your favorite foods again. Then ask yourself, "Am I hungry?" For most diet dropouts, that is a difficult question to answer. For other diet dropouts, the answer is always yes. In both cases, it is because diet dropouts aren't used to a having a healthy relationship with food. Expect to be frustrated as you're learning to answer the question and use this new rule.

More importantly don't forget to always preface the question by reminding yourself you will be eating only your favorite foods from now on. This is so you can start reversing all of those deprivation messages which have caused you to overeat.

Then, using the pleasure scale of 1 – 10, 10 being the most pleasurable, don't eat a meal or snack unless you feel it is going to rank between a 7 – 10 on the pleasure scale. The hungrier you are the higher eating will rank on the pleasure scale. Don't be too hard on yourself while trying to differentiate emotional and physical hunger. The New Rules honor both.

For example, let's say you know you're not physically hungry because you just had lunch, but you still would like to have a slice of the birthday cake your colleagues brought to the office for a fellow coworker. It's okay to join in the celebration and get a slice. But do apply what you can from the Rules #8 through #13.

You'll find that once you stop denying yourself and stop feeling guilty, a bite or two or three of that cake will be quite satisfying, instead of having to eat the whole slice. The New Rules honor the fact that food is very much a part of celebration and social activities - so let them eat cake!

Rule #8: Choose What to Eat with Your Pleasure Scale

Now this is where the New Rules get really fun! Aside from those exceptions such as food allergies and other medical implications, always choose the food you are craving! If you do have some allergy or medical restrictions, choose what you are craving within those confines.

This means every time you want to eat something, choose the food that is up near 10 on your pleasure scale! Remember: There are no more "shoulds" or "shouldn'ts". So if you are really craving apple pie ala mode for breakfast instead of your bran cereal, choose the apple pie! I am deadly serious!

I like nothing better than coffee, milk, and donuts in the morning and many, many, mornings of the last 15 years, I have had just that! Even if you want to eat potato chips for breakfast, lunch, and dinner, that's what you must do! Eat what you are truly craving at all times! And don't eat anything you think you 'should' be eating.

I know weight loss experts are writhing in opposition, but there are several reasons why this rule is so important. One of them is if you did choose the more healthy food over what you were craving, chances are very likely you will wind up overeating more healthy food to try and satisfy the original craving. But overeating is overeating regardless of nutritional content. The Simple Equation still applies: If you take in more calories than you expend, you will gain weight.

As discussed, our cravings are affected by so many things, some of them physical, some of them emotional, but they cannot be ignored. The backlash will come from a feeling of deprivation and it will cause us to overeat.

When first using the New Rules, chances are your cravings will come from the emotional issues the weight loss industry has plagued you with. You should actually expect you will be craving all those "forbidden" and "bad" foods you have been told you "shouldn't" be eating. That is exactly why you need to choose them to eat over and above other choices.

Once your brain is convinced these labels no longer apply to food, your cravings will come from a more balanced place. Your body will also be freed up to start telling you when it needs something more nutritious. But since the weight loss industry has tried to convince you to choose foods solely by your intellect, it will take some time to recognize your body's signals. It will tell you when it prefers an egg over a donut in the morning, but don't expect it to happen initially.

Of course, there will still always be those days when nothing else will do but French toast smothered in butter and powdered sugar, but you'll be able to see the more direct connection between your emotions and the food you're craving. And guess what? That is so okay!!!!

You'll probably also have more days that more healthy food choices are what you are craving. Even if that doesn't happen sooner than later, you'll still be taking your vitamins and drinking your water. You will also be enjoying the healthy benefits of guiltless pleasurable eating and the benefits of simply being thinner.

Usually later after using the New Rules for a while, you might find you really don't know what you're craving. That could be because you are truly not hungry. It could also mean the rules are so incorporated into your thinking food just really isn't that important anymore.

There are times during my day, especially while I'm writing or involved in something I am passionate about, I actually have to remind myself to eat! Can you imagine?! I certainly couldn't imagine forgetting to eat when I first began the New Rules!

But make no mistake - I still have those days when a handful of M&M's and popcorn along with a glass of wine is the only thing I'm craving! And that is exactly what I will have! I love these rules!

Rule #9: Eat the Best First

We've all heard the expression, "Leave the best for last." Like so many other misnomers, The New Rules turns that upside down. The New Rules say, "Eat the best first!"

For example, you order a steak dinner at a restaurant because you were craving steak. The dinner includes a salad with your favorite dressing and garlic bread, mashed potatoes with gravy, string beans, and the steak.

Using your pleasure scale, start giving everything on your plate a rating. What looks best? What rates a 10? What are you dying to sink your teeth into first? Then eat that first!

Also be aware parts of a certain food may rank more highly than the other parts. For instance, the center of the steak may be your favorite part so cut the steak in half and eat the middle first. You may rate the crust of the garlic bread more highly than the center so start by eating the crust. You love the bites of mashed potatoes with the gravy so start in the middle of the potatoes where the gravy is. Just start with the bites of everything that rank 10 and then move to the bites that rank 9 and then move to the bites that are an 8, etc..

Granted, this type of eating the best first isn't as pretty as starting from the outside in but there are benefits to that as well. I know when I order a cheeseburger in a restaurant, my favorite part is the middle. I'll cut the cheeseburger in quarters and eat the middle bites first. By the time I've eaten all the bites of the burger which rank over 6 on my pleasure scale, there is just scraps of bread with pieces of plain burger scattered amidst them with smears of ketchup and mustard. It's not very appealing but easily left on my plate, not on my waist!

But beware of your "Clean Your Plate Membership" here. It will definitely rear its ugly head if you're used to literally keeping your plate neat and clean. Which would you rather have - nice looking thighs or a nice looking plate?

If you've decided to forgo the more traditional choice for dinner, such as just skipping right to the dessert and ordering the peach cobbler ala mode, that's fine too. Eat the best of the cobbler first just as you would have the steak dinner.

The first time I did this at a restaurant while my friends ordered the more "normal" choices for dinner, you should have seen the reaction! You would have thought I had ordered illegal drugs!

"You can't have *that* for dinner!" was the unanimous cry at the table. All the usual diet mentality words came flying out of their mouths. However, I was the only one who left the restaurant perfectly satisfied. My friends were stuffed and complaining about how much they "shouldn't" have eaten!

Rule #9: Stop at Mid-Meal and Finish 2 Sentences

At the back of this book I have provided you with a *Jogging on a Dinner Plate Journal*. I've provided this for you because you are going to have to be your own coach. Ideally I would love to spend every meal with you for the next 30 days and coach you personally, but that would be very costly for you and there is only one of me to go around.

So, at every meal or snack I want you to stop at the halfway point of your meal and fill out the date and the first two prompt sentences in your journal:

I am really enjoying this ______________________.

I'm thinking about having ____________________

____________________________for my next meal.

It's not absolutely necessary, but try and go into a little bit of detail when filling out the first prompt such as "I am really enjoying this peach cobbler, because I love the crunchiness of the topping with the taste of the vanilla ice cream."

The purpose of the first prompt is to remind you to consciously enjoy every bite of what you are eating - something we have lost as diet dropouts. The purpose of the second prompt is to put your present meal into context, reminding you this is not a one-time occurrence. It is a reminder you will be eating something pleasurable at every meal - something your brain will not be willing to grasp very readily because of all the diet messages it has received.

Rule #10: Reassess Your Ratings

Filling out the prompts will give you a little time out from your meal. Timeouts are great because you can go back to your meal with your Pleasure Scale and reassess the ratings. Have the mashed potatoes cooled a little bit and most of the gravy is gone? They might rate a 4 or 5 now. The steak may still rate in the 7 or 8 area, etc..

It also gives you a chance to reevaluate your hunger level. Would you really feel deprived if you went ahead and left the rest of the meal and ordered the dessert now? Remember that even if nothing on the dessert menu appeals to you, you can go home and have some of your favorite cookies instead.

Rule #11: Stop Eating When Your Food Falls Below 6 or 7 on the Pleasure Scale

This is a rather self-explanatory rule. Again be patient with yourself while you are figuring out what falls below a 6 or 7 on your particular scale. I gave you a two-number leeway because it isn't necessary to be strict with yourself on this issue. Remember also emotional as well as physical factors are at work here so a 6 won't always look the same at every meal.

Don't forget - no one is ever going to take away your favorite foods again! With that in mind, if you are still hungry, certain foods on your dinner plate should still rate above a 6 or 7 on your pleasure scale. If not, don't bother. Leave it on your plate. You can always have something more pleasurable in an hour or two.

Rule #12: Leave at Least 3 Bites of Food on Your Plate

For some diet dropouts, it may be difficult to see anything on their plate as rating below a 6 or 7 initially. That was definitely the situation for me. If this is the case for you, just make the conscious decision to leave 3 bites of every food on your plate and 3 sips of every drink in your glass. This is one of those non-negotiable rules.

Believe it or not some of my clients have asked me how big a bite is. The answer is a simple one: A bite is as big as the bite you usually take. Can you see how entrenched people can be in the diet mentality? People are used to being told by the weight loss industry how big a serving or a portion is.

Now if you think you're going to outsmart the New Rules and leave 1 bite of something and cut it up into 3 pieces, you better think twice. Your body knows what you are doing! The amount of calories doesn't change by cutting it up in 3 pieces. And for those of you who are going to try that, I'm going to ask you to leave 9 bites instead!

As described in the chapter, *The New Rules are Born,* I used a salt shaker and poured salt over the leftover bites just so I wouldn't be tempted to clean my plate. Physically speaking, picking up the salt shaker is going to be the most laborious thing this program demands of you, but you must do it! You must leave food on your plate no matter what!

Rule # 13: Go Jogging on a Dinner Plate

Flip back to the page where you filled out your prompt sentences and then fill out the last sentences:

I left _________ bites on my plate.

_________ bites x ¼ = _________ miles that I ***do not*** have to jog to expend these calories.

So let's say you left 3 bites of steak, 6 bites of mashed potatoes, 5 bites of salad, 3 bites of garlic bread and 3 bites of green beans. Add them all together and you have a total of 20 bites of food on your plate that you would have ordinarily eaten.

Again, each bite of food is equal to a ¼ mile which you do not have to jog to expend those calories. Multiply 20 by ¼ and you get 5 miles that you ***do not*** have to jog! Which is easier - pouring salt over those bites of food or running 5 miles?

Rule # 14: At the End of the Day, Figure Out How Many Miles You Do Not Have to Jog

At the end of the day, right before you turn out the lights, add up all the miles you ***do not*** have to jog and literally dwell on it. Then congratulate yourself. Even if you didn't leave as many bites as you wanted, you still left some and they will ***not*** be stored up as fat on your body! Go to bed thinking about that accomplishment and also looking forward toward your breakfast tomorrow when again you will be having exactly what you want to eat!

Rule #15: Continue to Apply Rules #7 - #14 to Every Meal and Snack

Until you have a good grasp on the New Rules, carry this book and journal with you and continue to apply Rules #7 - #13 to everything you eat. Reread the chapters in Part I which really make a lot of sense to you. Continue to fill out the sentences in the journal. Eventually the New Rules will become part of your thinking and you won't need to use the journal or to reread parts of this book.

As days go by, consider leaving one or two more bites of your favorite foods than you did the day or two before. Your only goal is to continue to leave more and more bites on your plate until you are at the size you want to be and eating as much as your body needs to maintain that size. That's it.

You may be thinking, "Is that really it?" Yes, that's it. I told you it was simple!

The changes in your thinking about nutritional choices or exercising will all come into focus later. Those changes may or may not reflect those of other diet dropouts. They'll be yours - discovered and designed especially for you and by you not the weight loss industry.

Regardless, don't worry about any of that now. Simply apply these rules at every meal and remind yourself of the common sense points made in the Part I of this book. Then go on with your life. Before you realize it, you'll be a size smaller.

You'll be genuinely amazed at the subtle miracle which occurs by just applying these simple rules. "No Pain! No Gain!" will take on a whole new meaning for you. Once your weight is gone, then you can choose the pain of exercise and changing your food choices for health benefits - but again, only if you choose to. You do not have to do either to get and stay thin.

In an effort to make the implementation of the New Rules even easier, read *Part III: Frequently Asked Questions.*

PART III

Frequently Asked Questions

I truly believe I just have a slower metabolism than most thin people. Will the New Rules still work for me?

There are so many myths about metabolism. I can't tell you how many people have looked at me and said, "You obviously have a faster metabolism than I do." That is simply not true!

The fact is heavier people usually have a faster metabolism than thinner people because their bodies have to work harder. Additionally, the difference of metabolic rates between 2 people of the same approximate weight and age usually only differs by less than 3 percent.

Exercise can speed up your metabolism but even if the average person trained intensely for months to gain 5 pounds of muscle, that would only increase their metabolism by 2 or 3 percent. This only translates into being able to eat an approximate 30 – 40 extra calories a day! With the New Rules, you would only have to leave 2 extra bites on your plate a day to get the same weight loss benefits of an increased metabolism! So, yes the New Rules will work for you!

Additionally, as you become more in touch with your body signals through the New Rules, your body will tell you all about your particular metabolism. Your body will also tell you when and how to accommodate any changes in your metabolism.

If you want to take the much more difficult route of exercising regularly just so you can keep eating those extra few bites, that's up to you. But be aware that could easily throw you back into the whole weight loss mentality again.

I'm over 40 years old and I know that my metabolism has slowed down - that's when I gained all this weight. Isn't it unrealistic to think we can be the size we were when we were 20?

It's true your metabolism does steadily decline as you get older, but it doesn't change all at once on a particular day when your birthday cake has 40 candles on it. More importantly, your body knows your metabolism is slowing down. It knows it is taking fewer calories to fuel your activity.

But, again, people are so out of touch with their bodies they aren't letting their bodies do what they have to do to stay thin. Your body will tell you that you need fewer calories if you let it.

Assuming you were extremely active at age 20 and now you are not, yes, it is unrealistic to think you can consume the same amount of calories you did back then and not gain weight. But that applies to any age and at any time.

Remember the simple equation: To lose weight, you have to take in less than you expend. I was a size 18 when I was 20 and out of touch with my body and my food. I've been a size 4 for the last 15 years with the New Rules and obviously I'm 15 years older. So the answer to your question is it is not at all unrealistic to stay thin as we get older.

I know you said we shouldn't say food is good or bad, but some foods are really bad for your body and we shouldn't eat them, should we?

When I was trying to think of an analogy to this situation, I thought of the time when I lived in Los Angeles. If you live there you know that every day along with the weather report, you also get a report on air quality. Some days are just downright unhealthy to go outside and breathe. It is even recommended on certain days that people should not go out and exercise.

But the point is people don't move out of LA to breathe healthier air. Their lives and work are there and it is only realistic to deal with the situation and make the best of it. You don't see an entire multi-billion dollar industry trying to get people to move out of LA to a healthier city!

You can think about embarking on the New Rules in the same way. It's unrealistic to try and change your real choices and cravings at this point in time. The weight loss industry has unsuccessfully tried to do that for years. Instead, you must make the best of the present situation and still lose weight doing it.

So for most diet dropouts, it is important to consider food as more or less nutritional rather than "good" or "bad" for all the reasons discussed in the chapter, *Don't Hate Me Because I'm a Donut.*

After the New Rules have been wholly integrated into your life, you will be able to make healthier choices more often without feeling deprived.

Until then you must eat what you really crave and take your vitamins to pick up the slack.

The exception, of course, would be if you've been diagnosed with a medical condition. If eating peanuts will make your throat swell up and you would essentially suffocate, you would not eat them. If you knew you would die in a matter of hours breathing the air in LA, you would indeed move out of that city. It is only common sense to use the New Rules within the confines of any medical condition that you might have.

I've been using the New Rules for 2 weeks, and jogging an average of 10 miles a day on my plate, but I haven't lost any weight. What's up with that?

First of all, if you've stepped on a scale to find out you haven't lost any weight, you need to forget about continuing with the rules. Go find another unsuccessful diet and come back to the New Rules when you're ready to get rid of your scale for all the reasons explained in the chapter, *Changing Scales.*

If you suspect you haven't lost any weight because your clothes are fitting the same and you've been jogging 10 miles a day on your plate, you need to first congratulate yourself. If your clothes are fitting the same as they did 2 weeks ago then you have ***stopped*** gaining weight. And was it really that difficult?

You've been eating all your favorite foods and not had to really go jogging. Don't forget you would've had to actually jog 140 miles in the last two weeks to accomplish this same thing – stopping the weight gain. As described in the chapter *Last Notes,* you will probably lose weight more quickly toward the end of your journey with the New Rules.

You have 3 options to more quickly get to the phase where you are losing weight. #1: You can go find another ultimately unsuccessful fad diet. #2: You can opt to get a pair of running shoes and actually jog an extra 50-70 miles this week. #3: You can leave a few more bites on your plate at each meal this week than you did in the last 2 weeks, and continue increasing the number of bites left on your plate each week after that. Again, which is easier?

Don't ever forget what you leave on your plate you will not have to exercise off your body!

Instead of just leaving a few bites and increasing that over time, wouldn't it be better and quicker to just leave half of every meal on our plate?

Of course it would be quicker to lose weight if you left half of every meal on your plate. A few of my clients have been able to do that with much success. However, I don't encourage it because if you cut your consumption in half right away, chances are you will have physical hunger pangs.

You have to remember initially not only is your stomach physically stretched out beyond what it should be, your brain has also been stretched out in a way to consume a great deal of food. If you cut the consumption so drastically at first, chances are your body will object. More importantly your brain will tell you it's being deprived. And we know deprivation will cause us to overeat again.

**When I go out to eat,
I already leave about a half of
everything on my plate because the
portions are so big,
but I'm still overweight.
If I'm already jogging 10 miles
a meal on my plate,
How do I go jogging
during a meal like that?**

Hold on! The half of a meal you usually don't eat, doesn't count! The size of the meal you ordinarily eat is the one you go jogging with! If you are still overweight, those small meals are still too much fuel than you are expending.

You can't escape the simple equation. It applies to any meal you would try to fool yourself with by over ordering or over serving so you can log in a bunch of miles in your journal. If you're telling me you're logging a 1000 miles a day but you aren't losing weight, then I know you're fooling yourself, you know you're fooling yourself, and more importantly, your body certainly knows you're fooling yourself.

It also tells me you are probably treating the New Rules like the many diets you've been on before, by trying to "cheat". But you can't "cheat" the rules because they are based on the simple equation: To lose weight, you have to take in less than you expend. Nothing you can do can change that equation.

I know I'm overweight and it's hard to believe but I really do like diet soda over regular soda. Should I leave 3 or 4 sips of diet soda at every meal also?

I've said on many occasions that the New Rules try to instill common sense back into our eating. If you're drinking more than 6 diet sodas a day then yes, I would say leave 3 or 4 sips in your cup. It's not healthy to consume too much of any food - diet or not. But if it's a matter of having a diet soda or two a day, then I wouldn't worry about it.

In fact, if you truly do prefer some low-fat, diet, or sugar-free version of any food over the regular, go ahead and choose the healthier version to eat. However do make sure you truly prefer it over the other choice and you are not choosing it to lose weight faster. Your brain will interpret it as diet information and it will set you up for backlash eating.

Again, healthier choices will be made more easily once you've lost your weight and your brain doesn't interpret your choices as deprivation. Regardless, if the foods you do presently choose contain calories of any kind, do apply the rules and leave bites on your plate.

I know I can leave bites of food on my plate, but when it comes to my wine, I don't think I can leave 3 sips in that glass. What do you suggest?

Well, I can certainly understand because I'm a wine lover too! If you truly can't see yourself leaving 3 sips of wine or beer or other drink in your glass, then leave a few extra bites of something else you would ordinarily eat at your meal. And if you're going out for just drinks with friends after work, compensate for it somewhere else in the other meals in your day. You can trust yourself to be flexible with the rules.

I love McDonald's too and I usually drive through to get my food and eat it while driving. I've been told it's not a good idea to eat while doing things like driving or watching TV. What are your thoughts on this?

Like most things the weight loss industry has tried to tell us, I don't agree. I normally eat while watching television and often eat while driving. I believe this is part of the American lifestyle and we don't need to apologize for it. The theory is mindless overeating takes place while you are distracted. As discussed prior to this, I believe the causes for overeating start way before you plunk down in front of the TV.

Since the New Rules simply require you to leave some bites on your plate, the only thing you will have to adjust while eating and driving is to leave some food in the fast food bag. Of course, you won't be able to fill out the prompts in your journal so that should be done in your head and the bites logged later.

When I first used the New Rules while driving, I would take 3 or 4 bites of my cheeseburger and my fries and throw them in the rest of my unfinished drink. Trust me, you will not be tempted to touch your leftovers once they are drenched in soda!

You can use the rules while watching TV as long as you leave some bites on your plate. If you want to eat something like chips in front of the TV, don't take the whole bag. Put some chips in a bowl and then leave 3 chips. If you can't trust yourself to toss them before the commercial break, pour a little of what you're drinking over them. Soggy chips are very unappealing.

You talk a lot about backlash overeating and binges caused by the diet mentality, but I can't really relate to that because I've never really believed in diets. I do want to lose these extra 10 pounds though. Can the New Rules help me?

In a word, yes. The simple equation still applies to you. You need to take in fewer calories than you expend. If you are maintaining your present weight which includes 10 pounds more than you would like, you are currently consuming the exact amount of calories that you are expending.

Your options are similar to those of the diet dropout. You can buy a pair of running shoes and start running 20 miles a week or you can apply the New Rules and start leaving a few bites of everything you are presently eating on your plate. Which is easier?

I'm a guy. Whenever I have to lose pounds, I hit the gym. Are you saying I don't have to?

I'm married to a guy like you! My wonderful husband has gone up and down with his weight from the time he was a young boy and even into the time I've known him. Even though he seemed to understand and respect the New Rules, it took him a total of six years to REALLY get it.

That's why I want you to keep this book around because sometimes it takes a long time to really get it. What happened to him might happen to you. He tested the New Rules out a couple of times and they actually worked but then he would fall back into the diet mentality. He just couldn't really believe that he could lose and maintain his weight loss without hitting the gym and dieting.

Every other time in my husband's life when he lost weight it was because of exercise and diet. It was very difficult for him to disconnect the two. I'm happy to say he has been at one of his lowest weights ever for the past year. He still says to me, "I can't believe I didn't have to go to the gym!"

So many people who have known him at a much heftier weight now beg him to tell them his secret. He says, "It's my wife's program. I'll send you the book."

I think my problem is I'm a mom and I am pretty much making 3 meals a day for my family. I snack while I'm preparing those meals. How do I incorporate the New Rules into that situation?

I'm a mom too so I understand completely, especially when I make macaroni and cheese for my daughter. I love taking bites out of the pot right after I mix in the ingredients. Again, that is so okay. It doesn't fit in perfectly with the New Rules when it comes to leaving bites on your plate because usually you're eating out of a pot or off a cutting board.

Simply be aware you ate a good portion of your meal while you were preparing your family's meal and your body knows you did. So when you sit down with them serve yourself about half the amount you would have normally served yourself and enjoy! Do leave bites on your plate and still journal your food. It's just a matter of adjusting with a little common sense thrown in.

I know you say to leave at least 3 bites of every food you eat at every meal and snack you have, but what if it's a matter of a small cookie or candy shop chocolate? There are barely 2 bites to be eaten.

Eat half of the cookie or candy and toss the other half in the garbage, in the bushes, or any other place which is accessible to where you are. Food is biodegradable so don't feel badly about throwing it in the ocean or any other natural place.

I know it sounds silly to toss half a candy away but that is ¼ mile that you do not have to jog and you still were able to enjoy a taste of the candy! If you want to reach for another cookie or candy, do the same with that one, and the next one. That would be ¾ of a mile you will not have to jog!

I know that it is important to leave food on my plate to incorporate the New Rules into my life, but I really, REALLY hate to waste food. What can I do?

I suggest you reread and reread and reread the chapters, *Getting Your Money's Worth* and *Children and The Clean Plate Club*. If that's not enough, wrap up all the bites you've left on your plate and put them in the refrigerator. Maybe you can incorporate them in a meal later or perhaps give them to your cat or dog.

More than likely you'll forget about them so don't forget to clean out your refrigerator occasionally and remember - everything you toss in that waste basket didn't become waste on your waist!

If you are at a restaurant, ask for a doggie bag. As time goes on you will be surprised at how much you will be taking home. Anyone who has ever eaten in a restaurant in France or any other European country knows restaurant portions here in America are obscenely huge in comparison.

I was doing really great with the New Rules for the first 3 weeks. Then we went to an All-You-Can-Eat Sunday brunch and I totally blew it! I ate so many chocolate-covered strawberries I was sick as we drove home! Is this still the program for me?

Oh my gosh! I can't tell you how many times I've been there before! As I have said there are going to be times when you eat more than you would have liked but that is so okay! What is not okay is for you to panic and desert the New Rules.

You cannot "blow it" with the New Rules. Anytime you do stuff yourself, do not try to console yourself with promises of finding a really good diet that will really work "next time". You have solid scientific evidence and personal experience to know those promises do not work long term.

Instead, try not to think about anything until that horrible stomach ache is gone and then turn back to *Rule #5: Always Start Now!* The New Rules don't expect perfection. On the contrary, they EXPECT you to be human and overeat now and then.

I do recommend you avoid all-you-can-eat buffets as much as possible until the rules are completely integrated into your thinking for the very reasons stated in the chapter, *Getting Your Money's Worth.*

But let me share something personal about my life that will give you a glimpse into what kind of relationship you will have with food once the New Rules have done their job. My husband entertains on cruise ships for a good 10 months out of the year and I travel with him as much as possible. Because cruise ships are floating all-you-can-eat-buffets, statistics show the average cruise passenger will gain 8 pounds during a one week cruise!

One of the reasons I wrote this book was because of the many passengers who would question how I could stay so skinny while cruising so much. Delicious free food is literally available 24 hours a day on a cruise ship and passengers seem to want to get their money's worth in food alone while onboard.

My husband and I can thank the New Rules for keeping us thin while cruising or any other time for that matter. We both love food and because it is in its proper perspective in our lives, we get to enjoy any food onboard anytime we want without gaining a pound! It doesn't get any better than that!

The same is awaiting you, right here, right now. What do you really want to eat right now? Whatever it is, go get it and apply the New Rules!

Part IV

Jogging on a Dinner Plate Journal

DATE: ________

I am really enjoying this___________________________

____.

I'm thinking about having___________________________

____for my next snack/meal.

I left _________ bites on my plate.

________ bites x ¼ = _________ miles that I ***do not*** have to jog to expend these calories.

DATE: ________

I am really enjoying this___________________________

____.

I'm thinking about having___________________________

____for my next snack/meal.

I left _________ bites on my plate.

________ bites x ¼ = _________ miles that I ***do not*** have to jog to expend these calories.

DATE: ________

I am really enjoying this ____________________________

____.

I'm thinking about having ___________________________

____ for my next snack/meal.

I left _________ bites on my plate.

________ bites x ¼ = _________ miles that I ***do not*** have to jog to expend these calories.

DATE: ________

I am really enjoying this ____________________________

____.

I'm thinking about having ___________________________

____ for my next snack/meal.

I left _________ bites on my plate.

________ bites x ¼ = _________ miles that I ***do not*** have to jog to expend these calories.

DATE: ________

I am really enjoying this____________________________

____.

I'm thinking about having____________________________

____for my next snack/meal.

I left __________ bites on my plate.

_________ bites x ¼ = __________ miles that I ***do not*** have to jog to expend these calories.

DATE: ________

I am really enjoying this____________________________

____.

I'm thinking about having____________________________

____for my next snack/meal.

I left __________ bites on my plate.

_________ bites x ¼ = __________ miles that I ***do not*** have to jog to expend these calories.

DATE: ________

I am really enjoying this___________________________

____.

I'm thinking about having___________________________

____for my next snack/meal.

I left _________ bites on my plate.

________ bites x ¼ = _________ miles that I ***do not*** have to jog to expend these calories.

DATE: ________

I am really enjoying this___________________________

____.

I'm thinking about having___________________________

____for my next snack/meal.

I left _________ bites on my plate.

________ bites x ¼ = _________ miles that I ***do not*** have to jog to expend these calories.

DATE: ________

I am really enjoying this______________________________

____.

I'm thinking about having ____________________________

____for my next snack/meal.

I left _________ bites on my plate.

________ bites x ¼ = _________ miles that I ***do not*** have to jog to expend these calories.

DATE: ________

I am really enjoying this______________________________

____.

I'm thinking about having ____________________________

____for my next snack/meal.

I left _________ bites on my plate.

________ bites x ¼ = _________ miles that I ***do not*** have to jog to expend these calories.

DATE: ________

I am really enjoying this___________________________

____.

I'm thinking about having ___________________________

____for
my next snack/meal.

I left _________ bites on my plate.

________ bites x ¼ = _________ miles that I ***do not*** have to jog to expend these calories.

DATE: ________

I am really enjoying this___________________________

____.

I'm thinking about having ___________________________

____for
my next snack/meal.

I left _________ bites on my plate.

________ bites x ¼ = _________ miles that I ***do not*** have to jog to expend these calories.

DATE: ________

I am really enjoying this__________________________

____.

I'm thinking about having__________________________

____for my next snack/meal.

I left _________ bites on my plate.

________ bites x ¼ = _________ miles that I ***do not*** have to jog to expend these calories.

DATE: ________

I am really enjoying this__________________________

____.

I'm thinking about having__________________________

____for my next snack/meal.

I left _________ bites on my plate.

________ bites x ¼ = _________ miles that I ***do not*** have to jog to expend these calories.

DATE: ________

I am really enjoying this___________________________

____.

I'm thinking about having___________________________

____for my next snack/meal.

I left _________ bites on my plate.

________ bites x ¼ = _________ miles that I ***do not*** have to jog to expend these calories.

DATE: ________

I am really enjoying this___________________________

____.

I'm thinking about having___________________________

____for my next snack/meal.

I left _________ bites on my plate.

________ bites x ¼ = _________ miles that I ***do not*** have to jog to expend these calories.

DATE: ________

I am really enjoying this___________________________

____.

I'm thinking about having___________________________

____for my next snack/meal.

I left _________ bites on my plate.

________ bites x ¼ = _________ miles that I ***do not*** have to jog to expend these calories.

DATE: ________

I am really enjoying this___________________________

____.

I'm thinking about having___________________________

____for my next snack/meal.

I left _________ bites on my plate.

________ bites x ¼ = _________ miles that I ***do not*** have to jog to expend these calories.

DATE: ________

I am really enjoying this__________________________

____.

I'm thinking about having___________________________

____for my next snack/meal.

I left _________ bites on my plate.

________ bites x ¼ = _________ miles that I ***do not*** have to jog to expend these calories.

DATE: ________

I am really enjoying this__________________________

____.

I'm thinking about having___________________________

____for my next snack/meal.

I left _________ bites on my plate.

________ bites x ¼ = _________ miles that I ***do not*** have to jog to expend these calories.

DATE: ________

I am really enjoying this___________________________

____.

I'm thinking about having___________________________

____for my next snack/meal.

I left __________ bites on my plate.

________ bites x ¼ = _________ miles that I ***do not*** have to jog to expend these calories.

DATE: ________

I am really enjoying this___________________________

____.

I'm thinking about having___________________________

____for my next snack/meal.

I left __________ bites on my plate.

________ bites x ¼ = _________ miles that I ***do not*** have to jog to expend these calories.

DATE: _______

I am really enjoying this_______________________

____.

I'm thinking about having______________________

____for my next snack/meal.

I left ________ bites on my plate.

_______ bites x ¼ = ________ miles that I ***do not*** have to jog to expend these calories.

DATE: _______

I am really enjoying this_______________________

____.

I'm thinking about having______________________

____for my next snack/meal.

I left ________ bites on my plate.

_______ bites x ¼ = ________ miles that I ***do not*** have to jog to expend these calories.

DATE: ________

I am really enjoying this___________________________

____.

I'm thinking about having ___________________________

____for my next snack/meal.

I left _________ bites on my plate.

________ bites x ¼ = _________ miles that I ***do not*** have to jog to expend these calories.

DATE: ________

I am really enjoying this___________________________

____.

I'm thinking about having ___________________________

____for my next snack/meal.

I left _________ bites on my plate.

________ bites x ¼ = _________ miles that I ***do not*** have to jog to expend these calories.

DATE: ________

I am really enjoying this___________________________

____.

I'm thinking about having___________________________

____for my next snack/meal.

I left _________ bites on my plate.

________ bites x ¼ = _________ miles that I ***do not*** have to jog to expend these calories.

DATE: ________

I am really enjoying this___________________________

____.

I'm thinking about having___________________________

____for my next snack/meal.

I left _________ bites on my plate.

________ bites x ¼ = _________ miles that I ***do not*** have to jog to expend these calories.

DATE: ________

I am really enjoying this________________________

____.

I'm thinking about having________________________

______________________________________for my next snack/meal.

I left _________ bites on my plate.

________ bites x ¼ = _________ miles that I ***do not*** have to jog to expend these calories.

DATE: ________

I am really enjoying this________________________

____.

I'm thinking about having________________________

______________________________________for my next snack/meal.

I left _________ bites on my plate.

________ bites x ¼ = _________ miles that I ***do not*** have to jog to expend these calories.

DATE: ________

I am really enjoying this___________________________

____.

I'm thinking about having___________________________

____for my next snack/meal.

I left _________ bites on my plate.

________ bites x ¼ = _________ miles that I ***do not*** have to jog to expend these calories.

DATE: ________

I am really enjoying this___________________________

____.

I'm thinking about having___________________________

____for my next snack/meal.

I left _________ bites on my plate.

________ bites x ¼ = _________ miles that I ***do not*** have to jog to expend these calories.

DATE: ________

I am really enjoying this____________________________

____.

I'm thinking about having ____________________________

____for my next snack/meal.

I left __________ bites on my plate.

_________ bites x ¼ = __________ miles that I ***do not*** have to jog to expend these calories.

DATE: ________

I am really enjoying this____________________________

____.

I'm thinking about having ____________________________

____for my next snack/meal.

I left __________ bites on my plate.

_________ bites x ¼ = __________ miles that I ***do not*** have to jog to expend these calories.

DATE: ________

I am really enjoying this___________________________

____.

I'm thinking about having___________________________

____for my next snack/meal.

I left _________ bites on my plate.

________ bites x ¼ = _________ miles that I ***do not*** have to jog to expend these calories.

DATE: ________

I am really enjoying this___________________________

____.

I'm thinking about having___________________________

____for my next snack/meal.

I left _________ bites on my plate.

________ bites x ¼ = _________ miles that I ***do not*** have to jog to expend these calories.

DATE: ________

I am really enjoying this______________________________

____.

I'm thinking about having ______________________________

____for my next snack/meal.

I left __________ bites on my plate.

_________ bites x ¼ = __________ miles that I ***do not*** have to jog to expend these calories.

DATE: ________

I am really enjoying this______________________________

____.

I'm thinking about having ______________________________

____for my next snack/meal.

I left __________ bites on my plate.

_________ bites x ¼ = __________ miles that I ***do not*** have to jog to expend these calories.

DATE: ________

I am really enjoying this___________________________

____.

I'm thinking about having ___________________________

____for my next snack/meal.

I left _________ bites on my plate.

________ bites x ¼ = _________ miles that I ***do not*** have to jog to expend these calories.

DATE: ________

I am really enjoying this___________________________

____.

I'm thinking about having ___________________________

____for my next snack/meal.

I left _________ bites on my plate.

________ bites x ¼ = _________ miles that I ***do not*** have to jog to expend these calories.

DATE: ________

I am really enjoying this___________________________

____.

I'm thinking about having___________________________

____for my next snack/meal.

I left _________ bites on my plate.

________ bites x ¼ = _________ miles that I ***do not*** have to jog to expend these calories.

DATE: ________

I am really enjoying this___________________________

____.

I'm thinking about having___________________________

____for my next snack/meal.

I left _________ bites on my plate.

________ bites x ¼ = _________ miles that I ***do not*** have to jog to expend these calories.

DATE: ________

I am really enjoying this___________________________

____.

I'm thinking about having__________________________

____for
my next snack/meal.

I left _________ bites on my plate.

________ bites x ¼ = _________ miles that I ***do not*** have to jog to expend these calories.

DATE: ________

I am really enjoying this___________________________

____.

I'm thinking about having__________________________

____for
my next snack/meal.

I left _________ bites on my plate.

________ bites x ¼ = _________ miles that I ***do not*** have to jog to expend these calories.

DATE: ________

I am really enjoying this__________________________

____.

I'm thinking about having__________________________

____for my next snack/meal.

I left _________ bites on my plate.

________ bites x ¼ = _________ miles that I ***do not*** have to jog to expend these calories.

DATE: ________

I am really enjoying this__________________________

____.

I'm thinking about having__________________________

____for my next snack/meal.

I left _________ bites on my plate.

________ bites x ¼ = _________ miles that I ***do not*** have to jog to expend these calories.

DATE: ________

I am really enjoying this____________________________

____.

I'm thinking about having___________________________

____for my next snack/meal.

I left _________ bites on my plate.

________ bites x ¼ = _________ miles that I ***do not*** have to jog to expend these calories.

DATE: ________

I am really enjoying this____________________________

____.

I'm thinking about having___________________________

____for my next snack/meal.

I left _________ bites on my plate.

________ bites x ¼ = _________ miles that I ***do not*** have to jog to expend these calories.

DATE: ________

I am really enjoying this____________________________

____.

I'm thinking about having____________________________

____for my next snack/meal.

I left __________ bites on my plate.

________ bites x ¼ = __________ miles that I ***do not*** have to jog to expend these calories.

DATE: ________

I am really enjoying this____________________________

____.

I'm thinking about having____________________________

____for my next snack/meal.

I left __________ bites on my plate.

________ bites x ¼ = __________ miles that I ***do not*** have to jog to expend these calories.

DATE: ________

I am really enjoying this___________________________

____.

I'm thinking about having___________________________

____for my next snack/meal.

I left _________ bites on my plate.

________ bites x ¼ = _________ miles that I ***do not*** have to jog to expend these calories.

DATE: ________

I am really enjoying this___________________________

____.

I'm thinking about having___________________________

____for my next snack/meal.

I left _________ bites on my plate.

________ bites x ¼ = _________ miles that I ***do not*** have to jog to expend these calories.

DATE: ________

I am really enjoying this___________________________

____.

I'm thinking about having___________________________

____for my next snack/meal.

I left _________ bites on my plate.

________ bites x ¼ = _________ miles that I ***do not*** have to jog to expend these calories.

DATE: ________

I am really enjoying this___________________________

____.

I'm thinking about having___________________________

____for my next snack/meal.

I left _________ bites on my plate.

________ bites x ¼ = _________ miles that I ***do not*** have to jog to expend these calories.

DATE: _______

I am really enjoying this ____________________________

____.

I'm thinking about having ____________________________

____for my next snack/meal.

I left ________ bites on my plate.

________ bites x ¼ = ________ miles that I ***do not*** have to jog to expend these calories.

DATE: _______

I am really enjoying this ____________________________

____.

I'm thinking about having ____________________________

____for my next snack/meal.

I left ________ bites on my plate.

________ bites x ¼ = ________ miles that I ***do not*** have to jog to expend these calories.

DATE: ________

I am really enjoying this__________________________

____.

I'm thinking about having__________________________

____for my next snack/meal.

I left _________ bites on my plate.

________ bites x ¼ = _________ miles that I ***do not*** have to jog to expend these calories.

DATE: ________

I am really enjoying this__________________________

____.

I'm thinking about having__________________________

____for my next snack/meal.

I left _________ bites on my plate.

________ bites x ¼ = _________ miles that I ***do not*** have to jog to expend these calories.

DATE: ________

I am really enjoying this___________________________

____.

I'm thinking about having ___________________________

____for my next snack/meal.

I left _________ bites on my plate.

________ bites x ¼ = _________ miles that I ***do not*** have to jog to expend these calories.

DATE: ________

I am really enjoying this___________________________

____.

I'm thinking about having ___________________________

____for my next snack/meal.

I left _________ bites on my plate.

________ bites x ¼ = _________ miles that I ***do not*** have to jog to expend these calories.

DATE: ________

I am really enjoying this___________________________

____.

I'm thinking about having___________________________

____for my next snack/meal.

I left _________ bites on my plate.

________ bites x ¼ = _________ miles that I ***do not*** have to jog to expend these calories.

DATE: ________

I am really enjoying this___________________________

____.

I'm thinking about having___________________________

____for my next snack/meal.

I left _________ bites on my plate.

________ bites x ¼ = _________ miles that I ***do not*** have to jog to expend these calories.

DATE: ________

I am really enjoying this ______________________________

____.

I'm thinking about having ______________________________

____for my next snack/meal.

I left _________ bites on my plate.

________ bites x ¼ = _________ miles that I ***do not*** have to jog to expend these calories.

DATE: ________

I am really enjoying this ______________________________

____.

I'm thinking about having ______________________________

____for my next snack/meal.

I left _________ bites on my plate.

________ bites x ¼ = _________ miles that I ***do not*** have to jog to expend these calories.

DATE: ________

I am really enjoying this______________________________

____.

I'm thinking about having______________________________

____for my next snack/meal.

I left _________ bites on my plate.

_________ bites x ¼ = __________ miles that I ***do not*** have to jog to expend these calories.

DATE: ________

I am really enjoying this______________________________

____.

I'm thinking about having______________________________

____for my next snack/meal.

I left _________ bites on my plate.

_________ bites x ¼ = __________ miles that I ***do not*** have to jog to expend these calories.

DATE: ________

I am really enjoying this__________________________

____.

I'm thinking about having__________________________

____for my next snack/meal.

I left _________ bites on my plate.

________ bites x ¼ = _________ miles that I ***do not*** have to jog to expend these calories.

DATE: ________

I am really enjoying this__________________________

____.

I'm thinking about having__________________________

____for my next snack/meal.

I left _________ bites on my plate.

________ bites x ¼ = _________ miles that I ***do not*** have to jog to expend these calories.

DATE: ________

I am really enjoying this____________________________

____.

I'm thinking about having___________________________

____for my next snack/meal.

I left __________ bites on my plate.

_________ bites x ¼ = __________ miles that I ***do not*** have to jog to expend these calories.

DATE: ________

I am really enjoying this____________________________

____.

I'm thinking about having___________________________

____for my next snack/meal.

I left __________ bites on my plate.

_________ bites x ¼ = __________ miles that I ***do not*** have to jog to expend these calories.

DATE: ________

I am really enjoying this________________________________

____.

I'm thinking about having________________________________

____for
my next snack/meal.

I left __________ bites on my plate.

_________ bites x ¼ = __________ miles that I ***do not*** have
to jog to expend these calories.

DATE: ________

I am really enjoying this________________________________

____.

I'm thinking about having________________________________

____for
my next snack/meal.

I left __________ bites on my plate.

_________ bites x ¼ = __________ miles that I ***do not*** have
to jog to expend these calories.

DATE: ________

I am really enjoying this___________________________

____.

I'm thinking about having___________________________

____for my next snack/meal.

I left _________ bites on my plate.

________ bites x ¼ = _________ miles that I ***do not*** have to jog to expend these calories.

DATE: ________

I am really enjoying this___________________________

____.

I'm thinking about having___________________________

____for my next snack/meal.

I left _________ bites on my plate.

________ bites x ¼ = _________ miles that I ***do not*** have to jog to expend these calories.

DATE: ________

I am really enjoying this___________________________

____.

I'm thinking about having___________________________

____for my next snack/meal.

I left _________ bites on my plate.

________ bites x ¼ = _________ miles that I ***do not*** have to jog to expend these calories.

DATE: ________

I am really enjoying this___________________________

____.

I'm thinking about having___________________________

____for my next snack/meal.

I left _________ bites on my plate.

________ bites x ¼ = _________ miles that I ***do not*** have to jog to expend these calories.

DATE: ________

I am really enjoying this___________________________

____.

I'm thinking about having__________________________

____for my next snack/meal.

I left __________ bites on my plate.

_________ bites x ¼ = __________ miles that I ***do not*** have to jog to expend these calories.

DATE: ________

I am really enjoying this___________________________

____.

I'm thinking about having__________________________

____for my next snack/meal.

I left __________ bites on my plate.

_________ bites x ¼ = __________ miles that I ***do not*** have to jog to expend these calories.

DATE: ________

I am really enjoying this___________________________

____.

I'm thinking about having ___________________________

____for my next snack/meal.

I left _________ bites on my plate.

________ bites x ¼ = _________ miles that I ***do not*** have to jog to expend these calories.

DATE: ________

I am really enjoying this___________________________

____.

I'm thinking about having ___________________________

____for my next snack/meal.

I left _________ bites on my plate.

________ bites x ¼ = _________ miles that I ***do not*** have to jog to expend these calories.

DATE: ________

I am really enjoying this___________________________

____.

I'm thinking about having___________________________

____for my next snack/meal.

I left _________ bites on my plate.

________ bites x ¼ = _________ miles that I ***do not*** have to jog to expend these calories.

DATE: ________

I am really enjoying this___________________________

____.

I'm thinking about having___________________________

____for my next snack/meal.

I left _________ bites on my plate.

________ bites x ¼ = _________ miles that I ***do not*** have to jog to expend these calories.

DATE: ________

I am really enjoying this__________________________

____.

I'm thinking about having__________________________

____for my next snack/meal.

I left _________ bites on my plate.

________ bites x ¼ = _________ miles that I ***do not*** have to jog to expend these calories.

DATE: ________

I am really enjoying this__________________________

____.

I'm thinking about having__________________________

____for my next snack/meal.

I left _________ bites on my plate.

________ bites x ¼ = _________ miles that I ***do not*** have to jog to expend these calories.

DATE: ________

I am really enjoying this__________________________

____.

I'm thinking about having__________________________

____for my next snack/meal.

I left _________ bites on my plate.

________ bites x ¼ = _________ miles that I ***do not*** have to jog to expend these calories.

DATE: ________

I am really enjoying this__________________________

____.

I'm thinking about having__________________________

____for my next snack/meal.

I left _________ bites on my plate.

________ bites x ¼ = _________ miles that I ***do not*** have to jog to expend these calories.

DATE: ________

I am really enjoying this____________________________

____.

I'm thinking about having ___________________________

____for my next snack/meal.

I left _________ bites on my plate.

________ bites x ¼ = _________ miles that I ***do not*** have to jog to expend these calories.

DATE: ________

I am really enjoying this____________________________

____.

I'm thinking about having ___________________________

____for my next snack/meal.

I left _________ bites on my plate.

________ bites x ¼ = _________ miles that I ***do not*** have to jog to expend these calories.

DATE: ________

I am really enjoying this__________________________

____.

I'm thinking about having__________________________

____for my next snack/meal.

I left _________ bites on my plate.

________ bites x ¼ = _________ miles that I ***do not*** have to jog to expend these calories.

DATE: ________

I am really enjoying this__________________________

____.

I'm thinking about having__________________________

____for my next snack/meal.

I left _________ bites on my plate.

________ bites x ¼ = _________ miles that I ***do not*** have to jog to expend these calories.

DATE: ________

I am really enjoying this___________________________

____.

I'm thinking about having___________________________

____for my next snack/meal.

I left _________ bites on my plate.

________ bites x ¼ = _________ miles that I ***do not*** have to jog to expend these calories.

DATE: ________

I am really enjoying this___________________________

____.

I'm thinking about having___________________________

____for my next snack/meal.

I left _________ bites on my plate.

________ bites x ¼ = _________ miles that I ***do not*** have to jog to expend these calories.

DATE: ________

I am really enjoying this___________________________

____.

I'm thinking about having___________________________

____for my next snack/meal.

I left _________ bites on my plate.

________ bites x ¼ = _________ miles that I ***do not*** have to jog to expend these calories.

DATE: ________

I am really enjoying this___________________________

____.

I'm thinking about having___________________________

____for my next snack/meal.

I left _________ bites on my plate.

________ bites x ¼ = _________ miles that I ***do not*** have to jog to expend these calories.

DATE: ________

I am really enjoying this____________________________

____.

I'm thinking about having ___________________________

____for my next snack/meal.

I left _________ bites on my plate.

________ bites x ¼ = _________ miles that I ***do not*** have to jog to expend these calories.

DATE: ________

I am really enjoying this____________________________

____.

I'm thinking about having ___________________________

____for my next snack/meal.

I left _________ bites on my plate.

________ bites x ¼ = _________ miles that I ***do not*** have to jog to expend these calories.

DATE: ________

I am really enjoying this__________________________

____.

I'm thinking about having__________________________

____for my next snack/meal.

I left _________ bites on my plate.

________ bites x ¼ = _________ miles that I ***do not*** have to jog to expend these calories.

DATE: ________

I am really enjoying this__________________________

____.

I'm thinking about having__________________________

____for my next snack/meal.

I left _________ bites on my plate.

________ bites x ¼ = _________ miles that I ***do not*** have to jog to expend these calories.

DATE: ________

I am really enjoying this______________________________

____.

I'm thinking about having_____________________________

____for my next snack/meal.

I left _________ bites on my plate.

________ bites x ¼ = _________ miles that I ***do not*** have to jog to expend these calories.

DATE: ________

I am really enjoying this______________________________

____.

I'm thinking about having_____________________________

____for my next snack/meal.

I left _________ bites on my plate.

________ bites x ¼ = _________ miles that I ***do not*** have to jog to expend these calories.

DATE: ________

I am really enjoying this___________________________

____.

I'm thinking about having___________________________

____for my next snack/meal.

I left __________ bites on my plate.

_________ bites x ¼ = __________ miles that I ***do not*** have to jog to expend these calories.

DATE: ________

I am really enjoying this___________________________

____.

I'm thinking about having___________________________

____for my next snack/meal.

I left __________ bites on my plate.

_________ bites x ¼ = __________ miles that I ***do not*** have to jog to expend these calories.

DATE: ________

I am really enjoying this____________________________

____.

I'm thinking about having___________________________

____for my next snack/meal.

I left _________ bites on my plate.

________ bites x ¼ = _________ miles that I ***do not*** have to jog to expend these calories.

DATE: ________

I am really enjoying this____________________________

____.

I'm thinking about having___________________________

____for my next snack/meal.

I left _________ bites on my plate.

________ bites x ¼ = _________ miles that I ***do not*** have to jog to expend these calories.

DATE: ________

I am really enjoying this___________________________

____.

I'm thinking about having ___________________________

____for my next snack/meal.

I left _________ bites on my plate.

________ bites x ¼ = _________ miles that I ***do not*** have to jog to expend these calories.

DATE: ________

I am really enjoying this___________________________

____.

I'm thinking about having ___________________________

____for my next snack/meal.

I left _________ bites on my plate.

________ bites x ¼ = _________ miles that I ***do not*** have to jog to expend these calories.

DATE: ________

I am really enjoying this___________________________

____.

I'm thinking about having ___________________________

____for my next snack/meal.

I left _________ bites on my plate.

________ bites x ¼ = _________ miles that I ***do not*** have to jog to expend these calories.

DATE: ________

I am really enjoying this___________________________

____.

I'm thinking about having ___________________________

____for my next snack/meal.

I left _________ bites on my plate.

________ bites x ¼ = _________ miles that I ***do not*** have to jog to expend these calories.

DATE: ________

I am really enjoying this____________________________

____.

I'm thinking about having____________________________

____for
my next snack/meal.

I left _________ bites on my plate.

________ bites x ¼ = _________ miles that I ***do not*** have to jog to expend these calories.

DATE: ________

I am really enjoying this____________________________

____.

I'm thinking about having____________________________

____for
my next snack/meal.

I left _________ bites on my plate.

________ bites x ¼ = _________ miles that I ***do not*** have to jog to expend these calories.

DATE: ________

I am really enjoying this___________________________

____.

I'm thinking about having___________________________

____for my next snack/meal.

I left ________ bites on my plate.

________ bites x ¼ = _________ miles that I ***do not*** have to jog to expend these calories.

DATE: ________

I am really enjoying this___________________________

____.

I'm thinking about having___________________________

____for my next snack/meal.

I left ________ bites on my plate.

________ bites x ¼ = _________ miles that I ***do not*** have to jog to expend these calories.

DATE: ________

I am really enjoying this____________________________

____.

I'm thinking about having____________________________

____for my next snack/meal.

I left __________ bites on my plate.

_________ bites x ¼ = __________ miles that I ***do not*** have to jog to expend these calories.

DATE: ________

I am really enjoying this____________________________

____.

I'm thinking about having____________________________

____for my next snack/meal.

I left __________ bites on my plate.

_________ bites x ¼ = __________ miles that I ***do not*** have to jog to expend these calories.

DATE: ________

I am really enjoying this____________________________

____.

I'm thinking about having ___________________________

____for my next snack/meal.

I left _________ bites on my plate.

________ bites x ¼ = _________ miles that I ***do not*** have to jog to expend these calories.

DATE: ________

I am really enjoying this____________________________

____.

I'm thinking about having ___________________________

____for my next snack/meal.

I left _________ bites on my plate.

________ bites x ¼ = _________ miles that I ***do not*** have to jog to expend these calories.

DATE: ________

I am really enjoying this______________________________

____.

I'm thinking about having ____________________________

____for my next snack/meal.

I left _________ bites on my plate.

________ bites x ¼ = _________ miles that I ***do not*** have to jog to expend these calories.

DATE: ________

I am really enjoying this______________________________

____.

I'm thinking about having ____________________________

____for my next snack/meal.

I left _________ bites on my plate.

________ bites x ¼ = _________ miles that I ***do not*** have to jog to expend these calories.

DATE: ________

I am really enjoying this_______________________________

____.

I'm thinking about having_______________________________

____for my next snack/meal.

I left __________ bites on my plate.

_________ bites x ¼ = __________ miles that I ***do not*** have to jog to expend these calories.

DATE: ________

I am really enjoying this

____.

I'm thinking about having_______________________________

____for my next snack/meal.

I left __________ bites on my plate.

_________ bites x ¼ = __________ miles that I ***do not*** have to jog to expend these calories.

DATE: ________

I am really enjoying this______________________________

____.

I'm thinking about having ____________________________

____for my next snack/meal.

I left __________ bites on my plate.

_________ bites x ¼ = __________ miles that I ***do not*** have to jog to expend these calories.

DATE: ________

I am really enjoying this______________________________

____.

I'm thinking about having ____________________________

____for my next snack/meal.

I left __________ bites on my plate.

_________ bites x ¼ = __________ miles that I ***do not*** have to jog to expend these calories.

DATE: ________

I am really enjoying this___________________________

____.

I'm thinking about having __________________________

____for my next snack/meal.

I left _________ bites on my plate.

________ bites x ¼ = _________ miles that I ***do not*** have to jog to expend these calories.

DATE: ________

I am really enjoying this___________________________

____.

I'm thinking about having __________________________

____for my next snack/meal.

I left _________ bites on my plate.

________ bites x ¼ = _________ miles that I ***do not*** have to jog to expend these calories.

DATE: ________

I am really enjoying this_____________________________

____.

I'm thinking about having____________________________

____for
my next snack/meal.

I left __________ bites on my plate.

_________ bites x ¼ = __________ miles that I ***do not*** have to jog to expend these calories.

DATE: ________

I am really enjoying this_____________________________

____.

I'm thinking about having____________________________

____for
my next snack/meal.

I left __________ bites on my plate.

_________ bites x ¼ = __________ miles that I ***do not*** have to jog to expend these calories.

DATE: ________

I am really enjoying this___________________________

____.

I'm thinking about having ___________________________

____for my next snack/meal.

I left _________ bites on my plate.

________ bites x ¼ = _________ miles that I ***do not*** have to jog to expend these calories.

DATE: ________

I am really enjoying this___________________________

____.

I'm thinking about having ___________________________

____for my next snack/meal.

I left _________ bites on my plate.

________ bites x ¼ = _________ miles that I ***do not*** have to jog to expend these calories.

DATE: ________

I am really enjoying this____________________________

____.

I'm thinking about having ___________________________

____for my next snack/meal.

I left __________ bites on my plate.

_________ bites x ¼ = __________ miles that I ***do not*** have to jog to expend these calories.

DATE: ________

I am really enjoying this____________________________

____.

I'm thinking about having ___________________________

____for my next snack/meal.

I left __________ bites on my plate.

_________ bites x ¼ = __________ miles that I ***do not*** have to jog to expend these calories.

DATE: ________

I am really enjoying this__________________________

____.

I'm thinking about having__________________________

____for my next snack/meal.

I left _________ bites on my plate.

________ bites x ¼ = _________ miles that I ***do not*** have to jog to expend these calories.

DATE: ________

I am really enjoying this__________________________

____.

I'm thinking about having__________________________

____for my next snack/meal.

I left _________ bites on my plate.

________ bites x ¼ = _________ miles that I ***do not*** have to jog to expend these calories.

DATE: ________

I am really enjoying this______________________________

____.

I'm thinking about having______________________________

____for my next snack/meal.

I left _________ bites on my plate.

________ bites x ¼ = _________ miles that I ***do not*** have to jog to expend these calories.

DATE: ________

I am really enjoying this______________________________

____.

I'm thinking about having______________________________

____for my next snack/meal.

I left _________ bites on my plate.

________ bites x ¼ = _________ miles that I ***do not*** have to jog to expend these calories.

DATE: ________

I am really enjoying this___________________________

____.

I'm thinking about having ___________________________

____for my next snack/meal.

I left _________ bites on my plate.

________ bites x ¼ = _________ miles that I ***do not*** have to jog to expend these calories.

DATE: ________

I am really enjoying this___________________________

____.

I'm thinking about having ___________________________

____for my next snack/meal.

I left _________ bites on my plate.

________ bites x ¼ = _________ miles that I ***do not*** have to jog to expend these calories.

Easy Order Form

Each book is $14.95. Shipping and handling is $2.95 for the first copy and $1.00 for any additional copy. Florida residents please add 7% sales tax per copy ($1.05).

For credit card purchases:
Or call:

Revised Contact Info:
Susanna H. Dee
www.TheDonutWhisperer.com
TheDonutWhisperer@gmail.com

For check or money order purchases send this form to:

Susanna H. Wermuth
P.O. Box 752
Gotha, FL 34734

Please send me ______ books at $16.95 each (includes shipping). Florida residents please add 7% sales tax per copy ($1.05).

Please send me more information on:

___Speaking/Seminars ___ Mailing Lists ___Consulting

Name: ____

Address: ____

City ____________________ State ______ Zip: ____________

Telephone: ____

Email Address:_____________________________________